THE Fast
Metabolism Diet
COOKBOOK

THE Fast Metabolism Diet
COOKBOOK

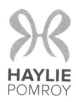

HAYLIE POMROY

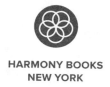

HARMONY BOOKS
NEW YORK

HAYLIE POMROY

The material in this book is for informational purposes only and not intended as a substitute for the advice and care of your physician. As with all new weight loss or weight maintenance regimes, the nutrition and fitness program described in this book should be followed only after first consulting with your physician to make sure it is appropriate for your individual circumstances. Keep in mind that nutritional needs vary from person to person, depending on age, sex, health status, and total diet. The author and the publisher expressly disclaim responsibility for any adverse effects that may result from the use or application of the information contained in this book.

Published in the United States by Harmony Books, an imprint of the Crown Publishing Group, a division of Random House LLC, a Penguin Random House Company, New York.
www.crownpublishing.com

Harmony Books is a registered trademark and the Circle colophon is a trademark of Random House LLC.

Library of Congress cataloging-in-publication data is available upon request.

ISBN 978-0-7704-3623-0
eBook ISBN 978-0-7704-3624-7

Printed in the United States of America

Book design by Ashley Tucker
Jacket design by Michael Nagin
Interior and jacket photography by Miki Duisterhof

10 9 8 7 6 5

First Edition

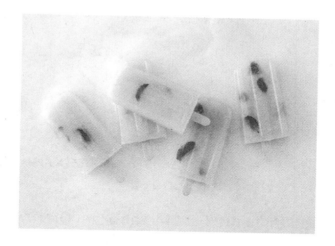

I dedicate this to my mother, Dr. Jeanne Wilson; my aunt, Pamela Chavez-Hutson; and my grandmother, Virginia Hutson, for their cooking made everything better.

CONTENTS

Part I: Getting Started

INTRODUCTION: Get Ready to Heal Your Metabolism with 28 Days of Delicious Food 9

CHAPTER ONE: What Is the Fast Metabolism Diet? A Recap 12

The Five Major Players 16
Your Pocket Guide 17
The Rules 20

CHAPTER TWO: Using *The Fast Metabolism Diet Cookbook* to Unwind, Unlock, and Unleash Your Way to a Thinner, Healthier You 23

A Guide to Portion Sizes 23
A Guide to Easy Food Swaps 28
A Simple Guide to Freezing and Crocking 29
Frequently Asked Questions 29
Planning Your Meals: 28 Days of Delicious Food 32

Part II: The Recipes

Phase 1

Breakfast 36

Lunch 42

Dinner 60

Snacks 75

Smoothies/ Beverages 80

Dips and Dressings 83

Desserts 86

Phase 1 Food List 89

Phase 2

Breakfast 92

Lunch 102

Dinner 115

Snacks 131

Smoothies/ Beverages 139

Dips and Dressings 142

Desserts 145

Phase 2 Food List 147

Phase 3

Breakfast 150

Lunch 162

Dinner 180

Snacks 191

Smoothies/ Beverages 198

Dips and Dressings 201

Desserts 204

Phase 3 Food List 207

Part III: Appendices

QUICK GUIDE TO VEGETARIAN AND VEGAN RECIPES 210

MASTER FOOD LIST 213

SAMPLE MEAL MAPS 218

BLANK MEAL MAPS 228

INDEX 236

PART I
Getting Started

Get Ready to Heal Your Metabolism with 28 Days of Delicious Food

If you've read *The Fast Metabolism Diet*, congratulations! You've just taken a huge step in repairing not only your metabolism, but your entire relationship with food—because the recipes in this book aren't just about repairing and or revving up a sluggish, slow, and burned-out metabolism (though they will). They are also about learning to love food again—relearning how to love its taste, its smells, its textures, and all the ways it nourishes your body and spirit.

I want you to let go of the death grip of fear food once had over you. I want you to learn to see food as your friend, your ally, your companion on your journey to a healthier, thinner you. I want you to relearn how to show love through the food you put on your family's table, and enjoy the love that your family puts into the food they cook for you.

You know the Fast Metabolism Diet is about eating, and it's about eating a lot. You know it's a diet that requires you to eat five times a day, sometimes more; that it's a diet about feeding your metabolism, using food to fuel your weight loss. But in order to do that you have to have real food, and real food needs to be cooked. And if you're as busy as most of my clients, that food needs to be easy, it needs to taste amazing, and it needs to be good for you. So this cookbook is all about learning how to cook food that tastes great, food that makes you feel great, and food that makes you look great: food that you can be proud to put on the dinner table for yourself, your guests, and your family. Cooking is about becoming an active participant in being well; it's what lets you take control of your health and repairing a metabolism that got broken somewhere along the way.

My family is fortunate enough to have a personal chef to cook all this delicious food—and that personal chef is me! Together we're going to turn you into your own personal chef—and the personal chef for your own family, friends, and loved ones—by teaching you how to create meals that strengthen your body, enhance your health, and light your metabolism on fire.

We are going to find the new you, and we're going to do it now. It's going to take a little work, but it's nothing you can't do. I'm not going to ask you to starve yourself ever again. That's likely what got you into this mess in the first place. So let's draw a line in the sand. If food has been your enemy in the past, that's all over. Now we're stepping into your future, where food is your medicine. It's the only thing we have to build our bodies, to create a healthy heart, strong bones and muscles, and good skin, hair, and nails. It's what we use to fuel the manufacture of hormones that regulate everything in our bodies. It's not just energy. It's life. It's time to stop being afraid to eat, and instead learn how to do it the right way. Whether you are ten or twenty or fifty pounds over-weight, you need this medicine. You need to learn how to use food to unwind stress, unlock fat, and unleash your metabolism.

I am out to revolutionize the way people feel about food, cooking, and the way they use food in their lives. That is why I've designed more than 250 nutritious, delicious, and easy-to-prepare meals that you can eat on all three phases of the Fast Metabolism Diet. It's why throughout the book you'll find lots of tips—some that I've come up with, and others that my clients shared with me—to help keep you on track as you rekindle your relationship with cooking, food, and weight loss.

But there are a few things you won't find in this cookbook. You won't find any fake or packaged ingredients. You won't find any artificial sweeteners or artificially sweet-ened foods. You also won't find any calorie or carb or fat gram counts. If you've read *The Fast Metabolism Diet*, then you know that "calories in, calories out" is a myth, and that I do not want you to ever count calories or carbs or fat grams. Instead, I want to see you cooking, preparing, and enjoying real food: the food that is the cornerstone of a healthy, fast metabolism. My primary goal is to promote health and make weight loss happen. It's what I do. It's who I am. And it's why we're going to get into the kitchen, together.

This is a diet full of pleasure, not denial. I am going to send you in a new direction, to help you enjoy food again, rather than fear it or deny it or portion it out on little tiny plates. With the Fast Metabolism Diet, unpleasant diet side effects simply aren't neces-sary. No starving allowed! You will shake up your metabolism in just the right way to increase your lean-muscle-to-fat ratio while enjoying improved health, more energy, and all the great food you're going to learn how to make in this book.

Cooking is a sacred and calming activity for me. At times, if you walk into my kitchen you'll find me with two slow cookers and a stock pot all going at once, because that's maybe the only night I have to cook for the entire week. After everything cools, you'll see Tupperware and freezer bags laid out all over the counter; after everything cools I portion it all out for family meals, one-serving meals, breakfasts, lunches, and dinners, and then I label everything and stick it in the freezer. It can be a crazy assembly line for one afternoon, but it makes the rest of the week totally seamless. Sometimes I even invite friends over for a bring-your-own-Tupperware cooking party.

But as much as I love to cook, I am also living a very full life and at times stretched very thin financially, emotionally, and for time, as I bet you are too. Therefore most of the recipes I have included are the things I prepare daily, so I know they are pretty quick and can be made on the fly. Many can be made on a shoestring budget; a few you could serve to a king. I also know that most of them freeze and reheat well.

These are all recipes I enjoy, and I cook them for my friends, family, and clients to enjoy too. In fact, many of them have given their input as to which favorites they wanted me to include. In more ways than one, cooking food creates community, and now you're part of that community, too. So in a way we will be cooking together. Know that I am most likely chopping, freezing, slow-cooking, and baking along with you.

So if you want to share recipes of your own, please visit my web site at www.fast metabolismdiet.com.

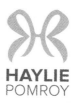

HAYLIE
POMROY

What Is the Fast Metabolism Diet? A Recap

Before we get into the kitchen, let's take a few minutes to recap what metabolism is, how it works, and why it got so messed up in the first place.

So what is metabolism, exactly? First, metabolism is a process, not an object. Specifically, the metabolic process consists of chemical reactions that occur in the cells of all living organisms to sustain life. It's the change or transformation of food into either heat and fuel or substance (muscle, fat, blood, bone). At any given moment, your metabolism is either burning, storing, or building.

You have a metabolism because you are alive, and life requires energy. We all need energy to survive—to breathe, move, think, and react—and the only way to acquire this energy is from food. Food that you have shopped for, chopped, cooked, and enjoyed. Profound! A healthy, functional metabolism allows us to have the perfect amount of energy available, an appropriate amount of reserve energy stored and ready for use, and a strong and stable structure (the body).

But an unhealthy metabolism, a slow metabolism, can't efficiently access the fuel from the food you eat, so instead of burning that fuel as energy, it stores it as fat on your body, saving it for a time when your body is in a healthier state. Dieting, nutrient-void foods, hormone imbalances, consuming chemicals and industrial pollutants mislabeled in the name of food, and living with too much stress are what slow down your metabolism when it should be sped up.

You may have tried a few or a few dozen diets in the past. You may have counted calories and fat grams or eaten packaged foods that had a shelf life of a million years. You may be frustrated with diets because you just can't stand to eat another fake cookie or disgusting bar or some artificially flavored and sweetened diet product all in the name of losing weight. Maybe you are even angry about investing time and money in a program that didn't account for the fact that you are a real person with real demands and needs and desires. Or maybe you lost weight but never repaired your metabolism, so the second you went off plan the weight came aggressively back. Maybe you are mad because you were never taught to shop for and prepare and cook healthy foods for yourself. We're about to change all that.

It's time to move beyond blame and regret and self-loathing, and into the future. This is the paradigm shift your body needs, and it will create a new, healthier version of you. The new you will view food as a tool to repair damage and restore health, and you will see the process of preparing and eating food as a joy and a cause for bragging rights. So many of my clients take pictures of the dishes they have made and post them on my Facebook page; many even drop the food by my office. Why? Because they are proud of what they cooked! My clients have fallen back in love with food, and so will you as you progress through this cookbook.

The new you will love fruits and grains and protein and healthy fats. If you've read *The Fast Metabolism Diet*, the new you knows how the body reacts to specific foods and strategic eating, and if you've picked up this cookbook, now the new you has all of the recipes and resources to cook all the food that's vital to get the weight off and keep it off for good!

Chronic dieting burns out your metabolism, but the Fast Metabolism Diet stokes the fires again. It works on a simple premise: confuse it to lose it. Just as you might cross-train your physical body to improve your athletic performance, cross-training your metabolism stimulates different burn, build, and restore mechanisms to maximize your efforts.

When your metabolism has become dysfunctional, it needs the equivalent of a personal trainer to get it back into shape—someone who can take food and use it to sculpt the raw materials of your body into the body of your dreams. Consider me that trainer and the recipes in *The Fast Metabolism Diet Cookbook* your guide to help you do it.

Think about it this way. If you do only one kind of exercise, such as running or using the elliptical trainer, your body gets used to that exercise and you soon stop seeing results. You hit a plateau because you're using the same muscles in the same way every day and neglecting all the other muscles in your body. In the same way that cross-training shakes up that routine by keeping your body surprised, the Fast Metabolism Diet shakes up your dietary patterns by flooding you with some of the vital nutrients you've been missing, but never in the same way for more than two or three days in a row.

This strategy keeps your body working, surprised, and supported, reversing the biochemical patterns that have slowed down your metabolism. It's your body's wake-up call, and it will trigger a burn that will torch calories and fat like never before.

Cross-training your metabolism also has the advantage of switching up the meals you're cooking and eating so your palate will never get in a rut or get bored. Two days eating one way, two days eating another, and then three days eating a whole new, delicious way. It's fun, it's interesting, it's delicious—and it works.

Remember, your metabolism is your body's system for dealing with the energy you take in through food. The metabolism shuttles that energy into different directions according to what you eat and what you do. The beauty of your metabolism is that it can be manipulated, because how you eat and move and live affects how much of your food is stored as fat, how much is used as energy, and how much is devoted to building the structure that is your body.

This manipulation is what I learned about when I studied animal science. The animal science industry uses this knowledge of energy, storage, and structure to create livestock that is ideally proportioned for use as food, to the tune of billions of dollars of profit.

Years of study and clinical work have taught me how to get your metabolism to stand up and pay attention, and how to push it to get busy and start burning away the fat that has plagued you for years. In this cookbook, I'll show you how to prepare the delicious and nutritious foods that will make it happen for you. I'm your nutritionist/personal chef now. With this book, I am bringing my program to you. I want everyone who wants to lose weight and get healthy to be able to do it—fast, effectively, and permanently.

This is not an eating plan for first-time dieters. This is an eating plan for last-time dieters. If you are about to give up on ever reaching your ideal weight, your battle is over. It is time to love food and know how to use it to bring about real, lasting weight loss.

Through my systematic rotation of targeted foods on specific days, at strategic times, the body transforms itself by cycling between rest and active recovery of the metabolism.

Your body stays surprised, nourished, and revitalized, until it becomes a fat-burning wildfire and the weight finally drops off the way you always dreamed it could.

You will eat in three different ways each week—according to Phase 1, Phase 2, and Phase 3. This phase rotation continues for four weeks, the same way every week, in order to cover every possible biochemical scenario in your body's monthly cycle (that goes for women and men). As a result, you'll start burning through food and scavenging body fat like never before.

This is not an empty promise. You can do this. I've seen it happen time and time again, for women, for men, for people in their twenties and those in their seventies. I've seen it happen for people in every eating population: people who are gluten sensitive, vegetarians and vegans, and meat lovers. No matter what foods you love to eat, this cookbook has something for you. The recipes are easy to follow and hard to resist.

In my clinical practice I work with a lot of clients with a lot of different eating restrictions, some prescribed by their doctor because of high cholesterol or because of a medical condition such as celiac disease or allergies. Others are due to personal preferences or ethical beliefs, such as vegetarianism or veganism. Because I'm in the clinical setting, I've had to develop foods and recipes tailored to all kinds of different medical and philosophical needs. That's why this book contains so many recipes that are easily adapted or converted to vegetarian or vegan (while still allowing you to add ingredients like buffalo or turkey or chicken to the vegetarian recipes, in case you prefer animal protein). It's why most of the recipes use alternative grains and don't contain gluten (the exception being the few recipes where I've noted that I use barley). And it's why all these recipes allow you to swap out any ingredient within the same phase and food group—so someone allergic to shellfish can swap scallops for halibut, or someone allergic to tomato can swap those beefsteaks for zucchini.

These recipes are actually favorites of many of my clients, many of whom have celiac disease, are vegetarian, or have severe food allergies. These are recipes carefully constructed for real people to introduce into their real lives. And now I'm so excited to be introducing them to you.

The Five Major Players

As you know, I view food as medicine, so let's do a recap of how you'll be using all this food to heal your body.

1. YOUR LIVER: The liver is responsible for more than 600 metabolic functions in the body each and every day. The liver regulates whether you store sugar as fat or burn it as fuel. Foods high in protein and nitrogen-rich alkalizing green vegetables such as those found in Phase 2 are catalysts for the liver's function.

2. YOUR ADRENALS: The adrenals regulate stress hormones, dictate muscle and fat development, and help keep blood sugar stable throughout the day. They are responsible for everything from your energy level to your mood level and are soothed and nurtured by high-glycemic fruit such as mangos and pineapples, and complex grains like brown rice and quinoa that you'll be eating a lot of in Phase 1. Thanks to the adrenals, the right foods can be one of the best forms of stress reduction.

3. YOUR THYROID: This metabolic rock star is responsible for more than 80 percent of your fat-burning ability. The hormones secreted by the thyroid are fed by the healthy fats found in avocados, nuts, seeds, coconut, and olive and grapeseed oil that you'll get to enjoy in Phase 3.

4. YOUR PITUITARY: The pituitary is the conductor of this amazing orchestra we call your body. It is vitalized by micronutrients in real live nutrient-dense, natural foods, the very essence of the Fast Metabolism Diet, and all of the recipes you'll find in this book have been intentionally put together to feed this conductor like a king.

5. YOUR BODY SUBSTANCE: You know the good old saying "You are what you eat"? It's 100 percent true. Your bones, hair, skin, nails, fat, and muscle structure are all dictated by what you eat, how the body metabolizes those nutrients, and how hormones regulate where you distribute those nutrients. These Fast Metabolism Diet recipes are all designed to build muscle, burn fat, and support healthy hair, skin, and nails.

Your Pocket Guide

You will cycle through three distinct phases for each of the four weeks of the Fast Metabolism Diet:

Phase 1—**Unwind Stress and Calm the Adrenals**
MONDAY–TUESDAY: **Lots of carbs and fruit**

Phase 2—**Unlock Fat Stores and Build Muscle**
WEDNESDAY–THURSDAY: **Lots of proteins and veggies**

Phase 3—**Unleash the Burn: Hormones, Heart, and Heat**
FRIDAY–SUNDAY: **All of the above, plus healthy fats and oils**

Let's consider how the three phases of the Fast Metabolism Diet coax your body to burn fat, build muscle, balance hormones, and lay the foundation for a healthier you. Our bodies require variety from our diets in order to get all of the nutrients necessary to perform all biological, physiological, and neurochemical functions. That's just what the three phases of the Fast Metabolism Diet give you. You need complex carbohydrates, natural sugars, protein, fat, and even salt to maintain normal body chemistry. At times you need very high therapeutic levels of these elements, especially when you've been depriving yourself for too long. Including these fuels, but not all at the same time, helps you to rebuild, restore, enrich, and replenish your depleted body and your burned-out metabolism.

Each phase lasts for only a short time so you don't exhaust any one system or part of yourself. Doing any phase for too long is like asking you to clean your whole house when you didn't get any sleep the night before.

For each of the four weeks, you will follow a three-phase rotation. Each phase is strategically designed to work and rest different body systems, and each has a chance to work during every week of your body's natural 28-day cycle. By segmenting out the work in this way, your body will get all the attention and support and high expectations it needs, one phase, or a couple of days, at a time.

So you are going to be cooking in three unique ways in one single week. On Monday and Tuesday you're going to be cooking for Phase 1; on Wednesday and Thursday you're going to be cooking for Phase 2; and on Friday, Saturday, and Sunday you're going to be cooking for Phase 3. Then you're going to repeat that weekly rotation four times for a total of 28 days. Each week consists of three unique styles of cooking, two unique groups of ingredients, and tons of variety. Because you're switching up what you're eating every two to three days, one week's worth of recipes could easily include fresh tropical fruit smoothies, hearty quinoa pastas, root veggie stir-fries, huge monster salads, comforting meatloaves, light fish dishes, creamy soups, and spicy chilies.

Phase 1—Unwind Stress

This is the high-glycemic, moderate-protein, low-fat phase.

HOW TO EAT

You don't have to start Phase 1 on a Monday, but I find this is the easiest way to stay organized. From the Master Food List for this phase, you will eat:

- **Three carb-rich, moderate-protein, low-fat meals**
- **Two fruit snacks**

See the complete food list at the end of this chapter.
Your day will look like this:

BREAKFAST	SNACK	LUNCH	SNACK	DINNER
Grain	Fruit	Grain	Fruit	Grain
Fruit		Protein		Protein
		Fruit		Veggie
		Veggie		

PHASE 1 EXERCISE

Do at least one day of vigorous cardio, such as running, the elliptical trainer, or an upbeat aerobic-based exercise class during Phase 1. Cardio is perfect for burning off excess adrenal stress hormones.

Phase 2—Unlock Fat Stores

This is the very high-protein, high-vegetable, low-carbohydrate, low-fat phase.

HOW TO EAT

If you started Phase 1 on Monday, then Phase 2 will always be on Wednesday and Thursday. From the Master Food List for this phase, you will eat:

- **Three high-protein, low-carb, low-fat meals**
- **Two protein snacks**

See the complete food list at the end of this chapter.
Your day will look like this:

BREAKFAST	SNACK	LUNCH	SNACK	DINNER
Protein	Protein	Protein	Protein	Protein
Veggie		Veggie		Veggie

PHASE 2 EXERCISE

Do at least one day of strength training (weight lifting) during Phase 2. Focus on lifting heavy weights with low reps. This stimulates the liver to lay down muscle and burn fat. Say good-bye to all that old fat that's been stored on your body for years.

Phase 3—Unleash the Burn

This is the high healthy-fat, moderate-carbohydrate, moderate-protein, low-glycemic fruit phase.

HOW TO EAT

If you started Phase 1 on Monday, then Phase 3 will always be on Friday, Saturday, and Sunday. From the Master Food List for this phase, you will eat:

- **Three meals**
- **Two healthy-fat snacks**

See the complete food list at the end of this chapter.

Your day will look like this:

BREAKFAST	SNACK	LUNCH	SNACK	DINNER
Fruit	Veggie	Fat/Protein	Veggie	Fat/Protein
Fat/Protein	Fat/Protein	Veggie	Fat/Protein	Veggie
Grain		Fruit		Optional: Grain
Veggie				

PHASE 3 EXERCISE

Do at least one day of stress-reducing activity such as yoga or deep breathing, or enjoy a massage during Phase 3. This will help support healthy hormone balance, including that superhero thyroid hormone.

The Rules

The food in this cookbook is so amazing, you may not have even noticed that we are following some strict rules. But our goal here is to repair your metabolism, so the rules are a must. Here they are; stick to them as you make my recipes your own.

So let's get cooking, because the first rule you're going to like: You have to eat. In fact, the number one rule on the Fast Metabolism Diet is that you have to eat five times, every single day. That's thirty-five times per week. And no cheating by skipping meals!

THE DO'S

RULE #1: You must eat five times a day. That's three meals and two snacks per day. No skipping.

RULE #2: You must eat every three to four hours, except when you're sleeping.

RULE #3: You must eat within thirty minutes of waking. Every day.

RULE #4: You must stay on the plan for the full 28 days.

RULE #5: You must stick to the foods allowed on your phase. Religiously. I repeat: Only the food list for your phase.

RULE #6: You must follow the phases in order.

RULE #7: You must drink half your body weight in fluid ounces of water every day (so for example, if you weigh 160 pounds, you have to drink 80 ounces of water).

RULE #8: You should eat organic whenever possible.

RULE #9: Meat choices must be nitrate-free.

RULE #10: You must exercise three times per week, according to your phase.

As you prepare your food, you will notice that a few ingredients are not included in any of the recipes in this book. They were left out intentionally; it was not a mistake.

THE DON'TS

RULE # 1: No wheat.

RULE #2: No corn.

RULE #3: No dairy.

RULE #4: No soy.

RULE #5: No refined sugar.

RULE #6: No caffeine.

RULE # 7: No alcohol.

RULE #8: No dried fruit or fruit juices.

RULE #9: No artificial sweeteners.

RULE #10: No fat-free "diet foods."

So whether you're cooking according to the letter of the recipes in this book or giving the recipes a twist of your own, do not try to sneak any of these ingredients in. I have left them out intentionally. These foods make it harder, if not impossible, to reset and repair the metabolism.

Remember, we've come together for a common goal. I am not here to be lenient; I am here to repair your metabolism. I can be tough when it comes to the plan, but it is tough love. I care about you. I care about your life and I care about your health. I'm here to help you and cook with you. All you have to do is eat the food—good food, delicious food, real food. In this book you'll find a huge variety of mouthwatering breakfasts, lunches, and dinners, as well as dozens of snacks, dips, smoothies, and even desserts that you can enjoy on each of the three phases of the Fast Metabolism Diet. You'll find countless vegetarian entrées and snacks, and over 75 filling and nutritious vegan options.

For my vegan friends I even added some soy-based proteins in a few of the Phase 2 recipes. Meat-eaters and vegetarians, these are not for you! Remember, only vegans get to break my no-soy rule, and only vegans may consume organic non-GMO soy products, and only on Phase 2! And even if you are vegan, I'm asking that you please use the soy sparingly because it is difficult to heal the metabolism and stimulate healthy fat-burning muscle with too much soy on board.

And here's more good news for the meat-free dieter: I've also included an easy guide to food swaps to help you make any entrée a vegetarian one—without losing the great taste or the nutrition.

You'll even find recipes for dips and dressings that can be eaten with any phase-appropriate meal; add 2 to 4 tablespoons to a salad, drizzle them over a filet, use as a marinade, or use them for dunking with any phase-appropriate raw or steamed veggies.

Confession: I love food! Sweet, salty, spicy, creamy, and tart. I believe that the pleasure of enjoying all kinds of flavors actually enhances your metabolism. That's why I've also included some delicious desserts and decadent smoothies that not only taste great, but when used strategically can increase the burn. So here's the deal:

BONUS RULE:

Enjoy Your Desserts and Smoothies in Three Ways . . .

1. Eat the dessert as a snack—as long as the treat includes the right phase-specific foods. It would look like this:

- In Phase 1: Eat any dessert that contains fruit. (example: Orange Sorbet page 88).

- In Phase 2: Eat any dessert that contains a protein. (example: Lemon Meringue, page 145)

- In Phase 3: Eat any dessert that contains healthy fats. (example: Coconut-Almond Pudding, page 204)

OR

2. Eat one additional metabolism-enhancing dessert with a meal— as long as it contains the phase-specific food groups for that meal, and you also add a day of exercise.

- In Phase 1: Add a dessert with a second day of cardio.

- In Phase 2: Add a dessert with a second day of strength training.

- In Phase 3: Add a dessert with a second day of stress-reducing activity.

So if you know you're going out for a special evening or you generally love something sweet before bed, just make that day your second day of exercise and enjoy!

3. Have a smoothie for any meal or snack as long as they fulfill the food group requirements for that phase.

- In Phase 1: Any smoothie that contains fruit and grain can count as a breakfast (example: Quinoa-Pear Smoothie, page 80), and any smoothie that's just fruit can count as a snack (example: Tropical Smoothie, page 82).

- In Phase 2: Since these smoothies all contain veggies, they can be eaten any time.

- In Phase 3: Any smoothie that contains healthy fat can count as a snack (example: Avocado Smoothie, page 198).

CHAPTER TWO

Using *The Fast Metabolism Diet Cookbook* to Unwind, Unlock, and Unleash Your Way to a Thinner, Healthier You

The Fast Metabolism Diet is a program designed to be tailored to your personal needs, your food preferences, your weight loss goals, and your lifestyle. So now let's use this cookbook to tailor the recipes and meal plans specifically to you. First up: portions.

A Guide to Portion Sizes

To figure out your portion sizes, first determine your goal weight. I'm not going to tell you what it is. You already know exactly how much you want to weigh and what weight makes you comfortable. Take that number and subtract it from your current weight. That number determines your portion sizes while you are on the Fast Metabolism Diet.

IF YOU HAVE 20 POUNDS OR FEWER TO LOSE: Go by the basic portions listed in the following table, and the portions included in the recipes in this book.

IF YOU HAVE 20–40 POUNDS TO LOSE: Add a half portion. For example, if a portion of soup is 2 cups, and you want to lose 30 or 40 pounds, then you would have 3 cups of soup.

IF YOUR LONG-TERM GOAL IS TO LOSE MORE THAN 40 POUNDS: Even if you have to lose more than 40 pounds, you'll be eating as if you only want to lose 40 pounds (for example, 3 cups of chili), with one exception: that is, I require that you double your veggie portion. So if the suggested portion for someone trying to lose 40 pounds is 2 cups of spinach, I want you to eat 4 cups of spinach so we keep our eye on the long-term goal and use that food as the catalyst for continued weight loss.

LONG-TERM WEIGHT LOSS GOAL: 20 POUNDS OR FEWER

	PHASE 1	PHASE 2	PHASE 3
Meat	4 ounces	4 ounces (2 ounces for snack)	4 ounces
Fish	6 ounces	6 ounces (3 ounces for snack)	6 ounces
Egg whites	3 egg whites	3 egg whites for meals, 1 egg white for snacks	1 whole egg plus up to 2 additional egg whites
Legumes/beans	½ cup	none	½ cup
Cooked grains: rice, pasta, quinoa	1 cup	none	½ cup
Crackers or pretzels	1 ounce	none	½ ounce
Bread, bagels, tortillas	1 slice bread, ½ bagel, 1 tortilla	none	1 slice bread, ½ bagel, 1 tortilla
Oats	½ cup uncooked, 1 cup cooked	none	¼ cup uncooked, ½ cup cooked
Fruit	1 cup or 1 piece	1 cup or 1 piece (lemons and limes only in this phase)	1 cup or 1 piece
Vegetables and salad greens	unlimited	unlimited	unlimited
Oils	none	none	3 tablespoons
Hummus	none	none	⅓ cup
Guacamole	none	none	⅓ cup
Avocado	none	none	½ avocado
Raw nuts	none	none	¼ cup

	PHASE 1	PHASE 2	PHASE 3
Raw nut and seed butters	none	none	2 tablespoons
Dressings	2 to 4 tablespoons	2 to 4 tablespoons	2 to 4 tablespoons
Smoothies	one 12-ounce glass	one 12-ounce glass	one 12-ounce glass
Herbs	unlimited	unlimited	unlimited
Spices	unlimited	unlimited	unlimited
Broths	unlimited	unlimited	unlimited
Condiments	unlimited	unlimited	unlimited

LONG-TERM WEIGHT LOSS GOAL: 20–40 POUNDS

	PHASE 1	PHASE 2	PHASE 3
Meat	6 ounces	6 ounces (3 ounces for snack)	6 ounces
Fish	9 ounces	9 ounces (4.5 ounces for snack)	9 ounces
Egg whites	4 egg whites	4 egg whites for meals, 2 egg whites for snacks	2 whole eggs plus up to 3 additional egg whites
Legumes/beans	¾ cup	none	¾ cup
Cooked grains: rice, pasta, quinoa	1½ cups	none	¾ cup
Crackers or pretzels	1½ ounces	none	¾ ounce
Bread, bagels, tortillas	1½ slices bread, ¾ bagel, 1½ tortillas	none	1½ slices bread, ¾ bagel, 1½ tortillas
Oats	1½ cups cooked	none	¾ cup cooked
Fruit	1½ cups or 1½ pieces	1½ cups or 1½ pieces (lemons and limes only in this phase)	1½ cups or 1½ pieces
Vegetables and salad greens	unlimited	unlimited	unlimited
Oils	none	none	4½ tablespoons
Hummus	none	none	½ cup

(continued)

	PHASE 1	PHASE 2	PHASE 3
Guacamole	none	none	½ cup
Avocado	none	none	¾ avocado
Raw nuts	none	none	⅜ cup
Raw nut and seed butters	none	none	3 tablespoons
Dressings	3 to 6 tablespoons	3 to 6 tablespoons	3 to 6 tablespoons
Smoothies	one 16-ounce glass	one 16-ounce glass	one 16-ounce glass
Herbs	unlimited	unlimited	unlimited
Spices	unlimited	unlimited	unlimited
Broths	unlimited	unlimited	unlimited
Condiments	unlimited	unlimited	unlimited

LONG-TERM WEIGHT LOSS GOAL: MORE THAN 40 POUNDS

	PHASE 1	PHASE 2	PHASE 3
Meat	6 ounces	6 ounces (3 ounces for snack)	6 ounces
Fish	9 ounces	9 ounces (4.5 ounces for snack)	9 ounces
Egg whites	4 egg whites	4 egg whites for meals, 2 egg whites for snacks	2 whole eggs plus up to 3 additional egg whites
Legumes/beans	¾ cup	none	¾ cup
Cooked grains: rice, pasta, quinoa	1½ cups	none	¾ cup
Crackers or pretzels	1½ ounces	none	¾ ounce
Bread, bagels, tortillas	1½ slices bread, ¾ bagel, 1½ tortillas	none	1½ slices bread, ¾ bagel, 1½ tortillas
Oats	1½ cups cooked	none	¾ cup cooked
Fruit	1½ cups or 1½ pieces	1½ cups or 1½ pieces	1½ cups or 1½ pieces
Vegetables and salad greens	unlimited, but double the suggested portions in the recipes	unlimited, but double the suggested portions in the recipes	unlimited, but double the suggested portions in the recipes

	PHASE 1	PHASE 2	PHASE 3
Oils	none	none	4½ tablespoons
Hummus	none	none	½ cup
Guacamole	none	none	½ cup
Avocado	none	none	¾ avocado
Raw nuts	none	none	⅜ cup
Raw nut and seed butters	none	none	3 tablespoons
Dressings	3 to 6 tablespoons	3 to 6 tablespoons	3 to 6 tablespoons
Smoothies	one 16-ounce glass	one 16-ounce glass	one 16-ounce glass
Herbs	unlimited	unlimited	unlimited
Spices	unlimited	unlimited	unlimited
Broths	unlimited	unlimited	unlimited
Condiments	unlimited	unlimited	unlimited

No matter how much you have to lose, you can eat as many vegetables as you want. But if your long-term goal is to lose more than 40 pounds, you need to eat at least *double* **the recommended portion of veggies with each meal and snack.** Still, when it comes to vegetables, the more the merrier. They contain all those important enzymes and phytochemicals that encourage fat metabolism, so have at it.

I get asked a lot about why I believe you need to eat larger portions when you have more weight to lose. If you begin this program with more than 20 pounds to lose, it's going to take more food (not less!) to keep your metabolism roaring. We're using food as medicine to heal your metabolism. If you walked into the doctor's office with alarmingly high blood pressure, the doctor most likely would put you on a very high dose of blood pressure medication to get things under control. He would then taper down the dose as the body stabilized. Well, when your metabolism is alarmingly out of balance and food is the medicine, you need to start with a high dose to get things under control.

And remember that no matter your portion size, don't hesitate to cook in bulk. These recipes are specifically designed to be doubled or tripled so you can freeze the leftover portions for the next time you cycle through that particular phase.

A Guide to Easy Food Swaps

Throughout this cookbook, you'll find lots of suggested food swaps to keep your palate revved up and excited. Some will be ideas for turning a recipe vegan or vegetarian; others will be simply to add even more variety to your diet. Do not be afraid to swap out one ingredient for another—as long as that ingredient is on the grocery list for your phase, of course

I typically tell my clients that if they make a particular recipe a lot they should try to swap one veggie for another veggie on the same phase grocery list, so their palate doesn't get bored. Just keep in mind that you can swap only within food groups: a fruit for a fruit, a veggie for a veggie, or a protein for a protein. I'm not saying you can switch your broccoli for pineapple; I'm saying instead of broccoli, try green beans. Don't think you can leave out chicken and replace it with brown rice. Instead, if you're in the mood for a vegetarian version, you can leave out the animal protein and replace it with lentils, black beans, or mushrooms (yes, I know this is a vegetable and I just told you no food group swapping, but this is one exception for vegetarians because mushrooms are so high in protein). Or say you are on Phase 1 and you want to make the buckwheat flapjacks, but you are allergic or do not like blackberries. Don't hesitate to swap the berries for mangos or Asian pears (both on the Phase 1 food list). Or, if a recipe calls for ground turkey and you prefer buffalo meat, swap away and enjoy.

You can also modify a food to fit into another phase (and you'll find lots of suggestions for these swaps throughout the cookbook, too). The other trick I have a lot of clients use is to repurpose their dinners into the next day's breakfast or lunch. For example, let's say you are on the first day of Phase 2. You make an amazing steak and asparagus for dinner and have some leftovers. Chop them up and scramble them with some egg whites for breakfast, or serve them over a bed of lettuce for the next day's Phase 2 lunch. Or let's say you are on the last night of Phase 2 and you have leftover halibut from dinner. The next day on Phase 3, chop it up, and add some safflower mayonnaise and sliced pink grapefruit for the best-ever halibut salad. Stuff this in an orange bell pepper and you have a lunch to die for! I also like to use my leftover brown rice from Phase 1 dinners and have it the next morning for a Phase 1 breakfast of a hot cereal with berries. Sometimes I take my Phase 1 chili and add diced avocados or some olive oil to make it into a Phase 3 chili. Or I take dinner from Phase 2 and add avocado or a hummus dressing on a bed of lettuce for a Phase 3 lunch. You get the idea.

At the end of the recipe sections for Phases 1, 2, and 3 you will find the food lists for each specific phase. Remember, ABSOLUTELY NO SWAPPING outside of your phase!

A Simple Guide to Freezing and Crocking

Here's a tip my clients have given me: In the first week when you will find yourself most motivated to cook, you should make large portions; label them Phase 1, Phase 2, and Phase 3; and freeze them so that you have them on hand for later weeks. I always suggest sitting down at the beginning of each week and filling in your meal map, planning the foods that you're going to eat for the whole week, and then creating a grocery list for all the ingredients you'll need. You might even consider repeating the exact same meal maps for week 1 and week 3, and week 2 and week 4.

Don't forget to make big batches of food and freeze for a later date. I like to label my frozen foods Phase 1, Phase 2, or Phase 3. This way I can just grab something on the go when I cycle through that phase again.

If you don't have a slow cooker or Crock-Pot I strongly suggest you get one. And, you can borrow another one or two more from a friend or neighbor (they probably have one they can dust off or pull out of the garage). I personally own three. One night a week, I make three separate meals—maybe I'll do Corned Beef Brisket and Cabbage, the Minestrone Soup, and Lentil Chili. All the prep and kitchen cleanup typically takes me less than an hour, then before I go to bed I turn everything on low and in the morning I have eighteen hot, delicious home-cooked meals waiting for me. I let them cool, portion them into Tupperware or freezer bags, label them for each phase, and stick them in the freezer to grab on the go when I have no time to cook.

Frequently Asked Questions

When I sit down to plan meals with my clients, I inevitably get a lot of questions, like "When can I eat these yummy desserts?" or "What spices can I use to give these recipes extra kick?" You'll probably have some of these questions too:

QUESTION: **When can I eat the desserts?**

ANSWER: Remember, on the Fast Metabolism Diet desserts are food. And, if placed strategically, they can be part of a fast metabolism. All the recipes in this book have been crafted to ignite your metabolism, so all the rules of the diet still apply to desserts. If the desserts fall into the correct categories for your phase-appropriate snack (like mango sorbet for a Phase 1 fruit snack), you can eat those desserts for one of your snacks. Also, if you want to eat dessert with your breakfasts, lunch, or dinner, you can do that if:

> · it meets the food requirements for that meal

> **AND**

> · you add an additional day of phase-appropriate exercise.

Please see my website, www.fastmetabolismdiet.com, for any further questions or examples on how to incorporate desserts into your lifestyle.

QUESTION: **When can I have the smoothies?**
ANSWER: Smoothies can count as a breakfast or snack as long as they fulfill the food group requirement for their phase.

QUESTION: **How can I eat the dips and dressings?**
ANSWER: You can eat any of the phase-appropriate dips or dressings at any of your meals or snacks. I typically tell my clients to limit the amount to 2 to 4 tablespoons per sitting.

QUESTION: **What if I like my dishes spicier?**
ANSWER: You can always add more herbs and spices. In fact, herbs and spices tend to stimulate digestion and enhance the metabolism. So don't be shy when it comes to turmeric or cayenne pepper. Basil, oregano, parsley, and cilantro are amazing to help reduce gas and bloat.

QUESTION: **They don't carry some of these ingredients in my grocery store. Where can I get them?**
ANSWER: A lot of the specialized grain products such as spelt, kamut or brown rice tortillas, or gluten-free breads can be found in the refrigerator or frozen section of your grocery store or health food store.

If you can't find an ingredient listed in one of these recipes, simply ask the grocer or the manager of your store to help you locate it. If they don't carry something, don't be afraid to ask them to special-order it for you; I have my local grocery store special-order things for me all the time, and they are always happy to do it (they may even give you case discounts if you're a frequent customer). Many of the items, like the coconut aminos, you can order directly from the company; many online retailers such as Amazon also carry those products.

If you can't find an ingredient in a recipe and you don't want to do a phase-appropriate swap (for example, if you can't find buffalo in your local grocery store to make my Buffalo Tip Salad and you don't want to swap it out with turkey), don't hesitate to try an online grocery store that will ship directly to your house.

QUESTION: What if I have eaten all my allotted food and am still hungry?

ANSWER: This question doesn't come often, but when it does, I have a sneaky feeling that it's because that client isn't eating enough vegetables. Remember, vegetables are unlimited; there's no reason why you can't snack on celery, radishes, cucumber, and jicama all day long. Make your lettuce or leafy green portion double or even triple if you find yourself still hungry. The fiber will help ignite the metabolism, stimulate your digestion, and give you those feel-full hormones.

The other thing you can do is drink hot teas, especially during the evening hours. The hot water is a natural vasodilator, meaning it expands the blood flow into the stomach, which stimulates feel-full hormones. So before you go for a second portion, try a cup of hot chamomile or peppermint tea. The feel-full hormones will be ignited by that temperature change in the stomach lining.

QUESTION: How do I cook without oil (in Phases 1 and 2)?

ANSWER: One of the questions I get often is, "How in the world do you sauté vegetables in Phases 1 and 2 when you're not allowed to use any oil?" I suggest you use products like coconut aminos or even a few tablespoons of vegetable broth instead of oil to stir-fry your vegetables. I use 2 to 4 tablespoons of vegetable broth for each serving of veggies. Just be sure to use slightly lower heat and know that your vegetables won't cook as quickly as they will when you're using grapeseed oil (which can get hotter, so it cooks your vegetables faster) in Phase 3. You can also cover your pan while sautéing vegetables, which helps soften them more quickly.

Another thing I like to do is throw my vegetables—especially root vegetables like carrots and sweet potatoes on Phase 1—in the slow cooker before I go to bed at night with just 1/2 cup of vegetable or chicken broth (no oil needed!) and they're ready when I wake up the next morning.

QUESTION: Can I drink anything other than water on this 28-day plan?

ANSWER: A lot of clients ask if they can drink anything other than water on this plan. The answer is that you can drink any unsweetened and non–artificially sweetened, non-caffeinated tea, but it doesn't count toward your total ounces that you need to drink for the day. So if you need to drink 100 ounces of water, you can have tea in addition to that but it has to be an herbal, noncaffeinated tea. Teas that are particularly hydrating are raspberry leaf tea and dandelion root tea; chamomile is exceptionally good to stimulate the liver, and peppermint is phenomenal for the digestion, especially during Phase 3 when you're trying to break down all those healthy fats.

QUESTION: **How many calories should I be eating each day on the Fast Metabolism Diet?**

ANSWER: Even after reading the book, people often still ask me how many calories, how many fat grams, and how many carbs they should they be striving for every day. I simply won't answer this question because it's about the nutrient density in the food, not the number of carbs or fat grams or calories you're consuming. Remember, it's the nutrients that activate the metabolism, not these things we like to think of as calories and fat grams and carbs. Fat comes in many different forms, and how the body processes it metabolically depends on the form it comes in.

QUESTION: **What if I have food allergies?**

ANSWER: Each phase of the Fast Metabolism Diet includes a very broad range of foods you can choose from, and the diet already excludes many common allergens, including wheat and dairy, so it's easy to cook meals around any food allergies. Also, since each phase is just two or three days long, you don't have to worry about getting bored with your meal choices.

QUESTION: **I'm vegan. Can I still cook on this diet?**

ANSWER: Yes, you can! For Phases 1 and 3, substitute 1/2 cup cooked, phase-specific legumes for meat. During Phase 2 (and only during Phase 2) you're allowed to break the no-soy rule in three ways to up your protein intake: tofu, soy tempeh, and edamame, as long as they're organic and non-GMO.

Planning Your Meals:
28 Days of Delicious Food

I wish that every single one of you reading this cookbook could come into my office and sit down with me and we could fill out these meal maps together. But since that's not possible, I've created the next best thing. There is an app I personally helped design to help act as your coach and nutritional counselor and help you plan out every day of eating on the Fast Metabolism Diet. You can use the app to create meal maps, track your meals and your water intake, and create grocery lists that you can even e-mail to yourself to help you get your shopping done.

To help you start planning your meals for the next 28 days with or without the app, there are sample meal maps from an actual client who had amazing success on the Fast Metabolism Diet.

You will see she swapped some of my ideas for her ideas and repurposed and converted some of her meals into new meals (always sticking to her phase, of course). In 28 short days she ate more food than ever before and lost more weight than she thought possible. And, as a bonus, I've added a fifth meal map with a week's worth of completely vegetarian meals so delicious that you'll never even miss the meat!

When you sit down to start planning your meals, you can either follow these sample meal maps to the letter, use them as inspiration, or flip through the cookbook, mark which recipes you'd like to try, and create your own original meal plan. As long as you're eating meals and recipes according to your phase, you're golden. And as you fill in your meal maps, don't forget that certain foods (see page 21 if you forget what these are) are off the menu completely for the next 28 days. And if it's not on the grocery list for your phase, don't eat it.

So follow my rules, take my recipes and make them your own, and in four weeks you'll be thinner and healthier than you ever imagined. And above all, remember: These are not just recipes for "a diet." They are recipes for a healthier, more delicious Fast Metabolism lifestyle.

PART II

The Recipes

PHASE 1

Breakfast

Creamy Brown Rice Cereal

Piping Hot Quinoa Cereal

Cinnamon Peaches on Toast

Buckwheat Flapjacks with Quick and Easy Blackberry Sauce

Apricot Tapioca

Sweet Potato Pancakes

Spicy Southwest Wild Rice Patties

Lunch

Sloppy Joe Turkey Wrap

Tangy Tuna and Veggie Sandwich

Toasted Bagel with Herbed White Bean Spread

Southwestern Burrito with Wilted Spinach and Bacon

Spinach Salad with Seared Pork and Squash

Tangerine Halibut Salad with Snow Peas and Mushrooms

Five-Bean Jicama Salad

Ice-Cold Gazpacho with Watermelon Chunks

Sweet Sausage and Cabbage Stew

Chicken and Sweet Potato Stew

Baked Italian-Style Beef with Winter Veggies

Mediterranean Turkey with Wild Rice

Black Bean–Arugula Wrap

Puréed Butternut Squash Soup

Slow-Cooked Minestrone Soup

Gingered Carrot-Orange Soup

Warm Steak Salad over a Bed of Spinach

Hawaiian Burgers

Dinner

Chicken Sausage Bowl

Tostada

Sweet Potato Shepherd's Pie

Halibut and Veggie Stir-Fry

Slow-Cooked Corned Beef and Cabbage

Stuffed Cornish Game Hens

Beef and Cabbage Wraps

Dover Sole with Tomato and Brown Rice

Broccoli and Fava Bean Stir-Fry

Pasta and Simmered Tomato-Meat Sauce

Garlic Chicken and Vegetables Over Quinoa

Ginger Pumpkin-Leek Soup

Sweet Potato and Broccoli Sauté

Vegetable Curry

Vegetarian Lentil Chili

Snacks

Cinnamon-Dusted Apple

Papaya with Lime Juice

Cucumber and Tangerine Salad

Chili-Kissed Mangos

Ginger Peaches

Grapefruit with Cinnamon

Minty Jicama Fruit Salad

Watermelon with Mint

Spicy Pomegranate Seeds

Smoothies/Beverages

Quinoa-Pear Smoothie

Three-Melon Smoothie with Mint

Green Apple Smoothie

Tropical Smoothie

Cantaloupe Smoothie

Dips and Dressings

Black Bean Cilantro Dip

Tangerine-Cucumber Dressing

White Bean–Dill Dip

Chunky Mango Salsa

Herbed White Bean Spread

Desserts

Quick Baked Apple Crisp

Mint Grilled Pineapple

Strawberry-Beet Sorbet

Orange Sorbet

Pumpkin Cookies

Creamy Brown Rice Cereal SERVES 1

PREP TIME: 5 minutes ▪ **TOTAL TIME:** 10 minutes

⅓ cup short-grain brown rice, uncooked

Dash of stevia

Pinch of ground cinnamon

1 cup Phase 1 berries

Put the rice into a blender and grind it. Bring 1½ cups water to a boil and sprinkle in the ground rice. Whisk continuously for 30 seconds and then only occasionally for 4 to 5 minutes longer, or until the mixture is thick and creamy and free of lumps. Sprinkle with stevia and cinnamon and top with the berries.

TIP: When I am in a hurry or have to make oatmeal on the go I love to dry blend it and turn it into a smoothie. It's like making my own protein powder!

Piping Hot Quinoa Cereal SERVES 1

PREP TIME: 5 minutes ▪ **TOTAL TIME:** 15 minutes

¼ cup quinoa, uncooked

1 cup fresh pineapple chunks

½ teaspoon ground cinnamon

Dash of stevia

Bring ½ cup water to a boil, add the quinoa, and simmer, covered, about 10 minutes, until water is absorbed. Top with pineapple, cinnamon, and stevia.

Cinnamon Peaches ✴ on Toast SERVES 1

PREP TIME: 2 minutes ▪ **TOTAL TIME:** 5 minutes

1 cup diced peaches

⅛ teaspoon ground cinnamon

Pinch of stevia

1 slice sprouted-grain bread, toasted

In a pan, mix the peaches with the cinnamon, stevia, and 1 tablespoon of water. Cook over medium heat until the peaches soften. Spoon the softened peaches and any syrup that collects in the pan over the toast and serve.

Buckwheat Flapjacks with Quick and Easy Blackberry Sauce SERVES 2 (1 SERVING IS 2 PANCAKES)

PREP TIME: 5 minutes ■ **TOTAL TIME:** 10 minutes

1 cup buckwheat flour

2 teaspoons baking powder

1 teaspoon cinnamon

½ teaspoon stevia, plus a pinch for the blackberry sauce

1 egg white, beaten

1 cup unsweetened rice milk

1 teaspoon vanilla extract

2 cups blackberries

Heat a nonstick griddle or pan over medium heat. Whisk together the flour, baking powder, cinnamon, and ½ teaspoon stevia. Add the egg white, milk, and vanilla and whisk well. Pour about ¼ cup of batter onto the hot griddle or pan for each of 4 pancakes and cook until bubbles begin to break on the surface. Flip the pancakes over and cook for about 30 seconds longer or until lightly brown. Meanwhile, heat the blackberries in a saucepan with ¼ cup water and a pinch of stevia. Pour the sauce over pancakes and serve.

Apricot Tapioca SERVES 4

PREP TIME: 5 minutes ■ **TOTAL TIME:** 10 minutes

½ cup small tapioca pearls

3 egg whites

⅓ cup xylitol

½ teaspoon vanilla

½ cup diced apricots

Any Phase 1 fruit

1. Add the tapioca and 1 cup of water to a medium pot. Let soak for 15 minutes, until most of the water is absorbed. Turn the stove to low heat and add an additional cup of water. Cook for 10 minutes and remove from the heat.

2. In a small bowl, whisk the egg whites, xylitol, and vanilla. Stir in 1 tablespoon of the hot tapioca to equalize the temperature between the two mixtures, and then stir the egg white mixture into the tapioca until evenly mixed. Add in the diced apricots. Serve warm or refrigerate and serve cold with a piece of Phase 1 fruit.

Sweet Potato * Pancakes SERVES 5 (1 SERVING IS 3 PANCAKES)

PREP TIME: 30 minutes ▪ **TOTAL TIME:** 30 minutes

1½ cups rice milk

1 cup cooked and mashed sweet potato

4 egg whites

1 teaspoon vanilla

1 cup brown rice flour

2 packets stevia

1 teaspoon baking powder

½ teaspoon cinnamon

¼ teaspoon nutmeg

Pinch of sea salt

1. In a large mixing bowl, whisk together the rice milk, sweet potato, egg whites, and vanilla. In a separate bowl, whisk together the remaining ingredients, and then whisk them into the wet ingredients.

2. Heat a nonstick pan over medium heat. Ladle the batter onto the hot pan by ¼-cupfuls and cook until golden brown on both sides, turning once.

Spicy Southwest Wild Rice Patties SERVES 1

PREP TIME: 5 minutes ▪ **TOTAL TIME:** 10 minutes

1 cup cooked wild rice (I use leftovers from dinners)

2 egg whites

¼ cup chopped Hatch green chiles

½ cup diced onion

Pinch of sea salt

Pinch of crushed red pepper flakes

1 piece Phase 1 fruit

Mix all ingredients together in a bowl. Shape into two patties and place them in a nonstick pan or skillet. Cook for approximately 2 minutes on each side until browned. Serve with Phase 1 fruit.

Sloppy Joe Turkey Wrap SERVES 1

PREP TIME: 10 minutes ▓ **TOTAL TIME:** 15 minutes

4 ounces ground turkey

⅓ cup diced tomato

¼ cup diced red onion

¼ teaspoon sea salt

¼ teaspoon fresh or dried oregano

1 teaspoon prepared mustard

1 brown rice tortilla

1 cup lettuce or arugula

1 cup chopped mango, pineapple, or any Phase 1 fruit

In a skillet over medium heat, brown the ground turkey with the tomatoes, onion, salt, and oregano. Spread the mustard on the tortilla. Lay a bed of lettuce on the tortilla and top with the ground turkey mixture. Serve with the Phase 1 fruit.

Tangy Tuna and Veggie Sandwich SERVES 1

PREP TIME: 5 minutes ■ **TOTAL TIME:** 5 minutes

6 ounces water-packed tuna, drained

¼ cup diced cucumber

2 tablespoons diced red bell pepper

2 tablespoons diced dill pickle

1 teaspoon prepared mustard

1 teaspoon balsamic vinegar

1 slice sprouted-grain bread, toasted

1 cup sliced apple, pear, or any Phase 1 fruit

Combine the tuna, cucumber, bell pepper, pickle, mustard, and vinegar in a bowl. Spread the tuna mixture onto the toasted bread. Serve with the fruit.

Toasted Bagel with Herbed White Bean Spread SERVES 1

PREP TIME: 5 minutes ■ **TOTAL TIME:** 5 minutes

- ½ kamut, spelt, or sprouted-grain bagel
- 2 to 4 tablespoons Herbed White Bean Spread (see page 85)

- 3 cucumber slices
  Handful of spinach
- 1 slice tomato
- 1 cup sliced apple, pear, or any Phase 1 fruit

Split in half and toast the bagel. Spread the bean spread on both halves of the bagel and top with cucumber, spinach, and tomato. Serve with the fruit.

Southwestern Burrito with Wilted Spinach and Bacon SERVES 1

PREP TIME: 5 minutes ■ TOTAL TIME: 10 minutes

1 slice cooked turkey bacon, diced

1 cup spinach

2 tablespoons diced red onion

2 tablespoons minced Hatch green chile

1 tablespoon organic vegetable broth

2 large egg whites or ⅓ cup liquid egg whites

1 sprouted-grain tortilla

1 cup Phase 1 fruit salad

Heat a nonstick pan over medium heat. Add the turkey bacon, spinach, onion, chile, and broth and cook for 1 minute, or until vegetables are soft and the spinach wilts. Add the egg whites and cook to the desired consistency. Wrap in the tortilla. Serve immediately with the fruit salad.

* Spinach Salad with Seared Pork and Squash SERVES 1

PREP TIME: 10 minutes ▪ **TOTAL TIME:** 30 minutes

4 ounces pork tenderloin, sliced in 1½-inch slices

1 tablespoon organic chicken broth

¼ cup sliced red onion

½ cup diced zucchini or yellow squash

Juice of ½ lime (1 tablespoon)

Pinch of crushed red pepper flakes

⅛ teaspoon sea salt

⅛ teaspoon chopped fresh cilantro

1 cup cooked quinoa

2 cups spinach

1 cup blueberries

Any Phase 1 dressing

In a medium nonstick skillet over medium heat, sear the pork slices for about 1 minute on each side. Remove from the pan and add the broth and onion and cook for about 2 minutes, stirring to prevent sticking. Add the zucchini and cook for 1 to 2 minutes or until the squash begins to soften. Return the pork slices to the pan and add the lime juice, pepper flakes, salt, and cilantro and cook for about 20 minutes or until the pork is cooked through and the zucchini is tender. Mix in the quinoa and heat for about 1 minute to make sure everything blends nicely. Serve over a bed of spinach. Garnish with the blueberries, dress with any Phase 1 dressing, and serve with remaining blueberries on the side.

Tangerine Halibut Salad with Snow Peas and Mushrooms SERVES 1

PREP TIME: 15 minutes ▪ **TOTAL TIME:** 25 minutes

½ cup shredded cabbage

½ cup snow peas

¼ cup sliced bamboo shoots

¼ cup diced green onion (scallions), white and green parts

¼ cup sliced mushrooms

1 tablespoon coconut aminos

Pinch of mustard seed

6 ounces cubed halibut

2 cups mixed salad greens

1 tangerine, peeled and sectioned

10 rice crackers, crumbled

Juice of ½ lime (1 tablespoon)

Any Phase 1 dressing

In a medium pot with a lid, combine the cabbage, snow peas, bamboo shoots, green onion, aminos, mushrooms, and mustard seeds. Cook, stirring often, for 3 minutes, until the vegetables are barely tender. Add the halibut, cover, and cook for 5 to 7 minutes, until the fish flakes easily with a fork. Remove from the heat. Place the halibut mixture on a bed of greens, top with tangerine sections, lime juice, crumbled rice crackers, and dress with any Phase 1 dressing.

Five-Bean Jicama Salad SERVES 12

PREP TIME: 10 minutes ■ **TOTAL TIME:** 45 minutes (includes 35 minutes for chilling)

1 15-ounce can white beans

1 15-ounce can black beans

1 15-ounce can kidney beans

1 15-ounce can garbanzo beans

1 cup cooked green beans6, cut up

½ cup chopped red onion

½ cup diced jicama

¾ cup organic vegetable broth

¾ cup red wine vinegar

¼ cup stevia or birch xylitol

¾ teaspoon dry mustard

½ teaspoon fresh or dried tarragon

½ teaspoon fresh or dried cilantro

2 cups wild rice, cooked

1 cup Phase 1 fruit salad per serving

Rinse and drain the white, black, kidney, garbanzo, and green beans and put them in a large mixing bowl. Add the onion and jicama and set aside. In a small saucepan, combine the vegetable broth, vinegar, stevia, mustard, tarragon, and cilantro. Cook over medium heat, stirring, for about 5 minutes, or until the stevia dissolves. If using xylitol, cook until dissolved. Pour over the bean mixture. Stir, cover, and refrigerate until chilled. Serve with wild rice and fruit salad on the side.

TIP: Because beans are both a protein and a starch, I like to add just a little wild rice to this dish to enhance the fat-burning carbs.

TIP: This is one of my favorite meals to bring to a potluck or party. It feeds a lot! And it pairs great with a Phase 1 fruit salad!

Ice-Cold Gazpacho with Watermelon Chunks SERVES 3

PREP TIME: 20 minutes ■ **TOTAL TIME:** 1 hour 20 minutes (includes 1 hour for chilling)

- **4 ripe medium-size tomatoes, peeled and chopped**
- **1½ cups organic vegetable broth**
- **1½ cups drained garbanzo beans**
- **1 celery stalk, chopped**
- **½ garlic clove, minced**
- **½ red onion, diced**
- **½ cucumber, diced**
- **½ red bell pepper, diced**
- **¼ cup tomato paste**
- **2 tablespoons red wine vinegar**
- **1 tablespoon chopped fresh parsley**
- **1 tablespoon chopped fresh chives**
- **1 tablespoon lemon juice**
- **1 teaspoon birch xylitol**
- **½ teaspoon crushed red pepper flakes**
- **½ teaspoon tamari**
- **Sea salt and black pepper**
- **3 cups cubed watermelon**
- **6 fresh mint leaves**
- **1½ cups spelt pretzels**

Combine all ingredients except the watermelon, mint, and pretzels in a blender (work in batches if necessary). Blend on low for 15 seconds. The soup should not be completely smooth but have some texture. Refrigerate for at least 1 hour and up to 12 hours before serving. Garnish each serving with diced watermelon and 2 mint leaves. Serve with ½ cup spelt pretzels for each serving.

Sweet Sausage and Cabbage Stew SERVES 6

PREP TIME: 10 minutes ▪ TOTAL TIME: 3 to 8 hours (slow cooker)

1½ pounds chicken sausage, sliced

6 green apples, cored and diced

6 cups shredded cabbage

1 cup diced onion

¾ cup organic chicken broth

⅓ cup birch xylitol

1 teaspoon sea salt

½ teaspoon black pepper

½ teaspoon ground nutmeg

¼ teaspoon ground cinnamon

1 fresh or dried bay leaf

6 cups cooked wild rice, rinsed

Put all ingredients except the rice in a slow cooker or Crock-Pot and cook for 3 to 4 hours on high or 6 to 8 hours on low. Remove the bay leaf, spoon the sausage stew over the cooked rice and serve.

Chicken and Sweet Potato Stew SERVES 6

PREP TIME: 10 minutes ▪ **TOTAL TIME:** 3 to 8 hours (slow cooker)

5 slices turkey bacon, chopped

1½ pounds boneless, skinless chicken breasts

½ cup organic chicken broth

⅔ cup sliced green onions (scallions), white and green parts

¼ pound mushrooms, sliced

4 sweet potatoes, cut into quarters

1 yellow onion, diced

½ cup uncooked quinoa or brown or wild rice

⅓ cup red wine vinegar

1 tablespoon minced garlic

1 teaspoon sea salt

½ teaspoon black pepper

½ teaspoon fresh thyme leaves

6 cups figs, kiwis, papaya, or any Phase 1 fruit

1. Heat a nonstick skillet over medium heat and cook the turkey bacon for about 5 minutes, until slightly browned. Remove the bacon from the pan and drain on paper towels. Add the chicken breasts and cook for 3 to 4 minutes or until browned on one side. Turn each breast over, add 2 tablespoons of the chicken broth, and cook for an additional 3 minutes.

2. Put the bacon and chicken in a slow cooker or Crock-Pot and then add the remaining ingredients, except the fruit. Cook for 3 to 4 hours on high or 6 to 8 hours on low. Serve the stew hot with 1 cup of the fruit per serving.

TIP: Because sweet potatoes also contain starch, I like to use a little less quinoa in this recipe to keep your body in burn, not storage mode.

Baked Italian-Style Beef with Winter Veggies SERVES 4

PREP TIME: 10 minutes ▪ **TOTAL TIME:** 1 hour 10 minutes

2 zucchini

2 yellow squash

4 4-ounce pieces steak

1 15-ounce can organic diced tomatoes*

1 teaspoon fresh or dried oregano

1 teaspoon minced garlic

1 large red onion, sliced

Sea salt and pepper to taste

4 cups cooked brown rice or brown rice pasta

1. Preheat the oven to 375°F.

2. Cut off the ends of the zucchini and yellow squash and shave the squash into long strips using a vegetable peeler. Place the pieces of steak in a nonstick baking dish and top with the squash strips. Combine the tomatoes with the oregano and garlic and then spoon the tomatoes over the squash. Lay the onion slices on top of the tomatoes and then cover with aluminum foil. Bake for about 1 hour, or until the meat is cooked to the desired degree of doneness. Season with salt and pepper to taste and serve with rice or pasta.

*Because tomatoes are cooked, which increases their glycemic value, and I put so much of them in this recipe, you can count them as your Phase 1 fruit.

Mediterranean Turkey with Wild Rice **SERVES 6 TO 8**

PREP TIME: 10 minutes ▪ **TOTAL TIME:** 3 to 8 hours (slow cooker)

4 large tomatoes, diced

4 cups diced zucchini

4 cups organic vegetable broth

2 cups uncooked wild rice

1½ to 2 pounds cubed turkey breast

½ cup sliced onion

¼ cup chopped fresh parsley

1 tablespoon minced garlic

1 tablespoon lemon juice

Put all ingredients into a slow cooker or Crock-Pot and cook for 3 to 4 hours on high or 6 to 8 hours on low. Serve hot.

Black Bean–Arugula Wrap SERVES 1

PREP TIME: 5 minutes ▪ TOTAL TIME: 5 minutes

1 brown rice tortilla

½ cup canned black beans, drained and rinsed

1 cup arugula

2 tablespoons diced red onion

½ cup diced tomato

1 teaspoon chopped fresh cilantro

¼ teaspoon chili powder

Juice of ¼ lime (1½ teaspoons)

1 cup blueberries, raspberries, or other Phase 1 fruit

Warm the tortilla on the stove or in a microwave. Spoon the black beans down the center of the tortilla and top with the arugula, onions, tomatoes, and cilantro. Sprinkle with the chili powder and then with the lime juice. Wrap the tortilla around the filling and eat with the fruit on the side.

Puréed Butternut Squash Soup SERVES 6

PREP TIME: 20 minutes ■ **TOTAL TIME:** 1 hour 10 minutes

1 large butternut squash

1 tablespoon sea salt

1 cup finely chopped white onion

3 garlic cloves, minced

5 cups organic vegetable or chicken broth

2 15-ounce cans black beans, drained and rinsed

1½ teaspoons caraway seeds

1 teaspoon black pepper

6 slices sprouted-grain bread, toasted, or 3 sprouted-grain bagels, split

6 cups chopped mango, pineapple, or any Phase 1 fruit

1. Preheat the oven to 375°F.

2. Cut the squash in half and remove the seeds. Set the halved squash on a baking sheet and fill the scooped-out cavities with water. Bake for 35 to 40 minutes, or until the flesh is tender when pierced with a fork or small knife. Scoop the flesh from the skin and transfer to a mixing bowl. Season with salt and stir until as smooth as possible.

3. Heat a deep nonstick skillet over medium-high heat and cook the onion and garlic, stirring often, for 5 to 8 minutes or until tender. Take care not to burn the garlic. Add the broth, beans, caraway seeds, and pepper. Bring to a boil, reduce the heat, and simmer for about 10 minutes. Add the squash and mix well.

4. Purée in a blender in batches until smooth. Transfer the soup to a large pot and heat gently until hot. Serve with a slice of toast or bagel and 1 cup of Phase 1 fruit per serving.

Slow-Cooked Minestrone Soup **SERVES 3**

PREP TIME: 10 minutes ▪ **TOTAL TIME:** 4 to 8 hours (slow cooker)

1 15-ounce can kidney beans, drained

4 cups organic vegetable broth

3 cups diced tomatoes*

1 cup sliced carrots

1 cup diced zucchini

1 cup shredded cabbage

1 red onion, diced

2 garlic cloves, minced

1 teaspoon fresh or dried basil

1 teaspoon fresh or dried parsley

½ teaspoon fresh or dried oregano

½ teaspoon sea salt

¼ teaspoon black pepper

3 cups cooked fusilli

Put all ingredients except the fusilli into a slow cooker or Crock-Pot and mix thoroughly. Cook for 4 to 6 hours on high or 6 to 8 hours on low. Add the cooked fusilli to the soup and serve.

*In this recipe the tomato can count as your Phase 1 fruit.

Gingered Carrot-Orange Soup SERVES 6

PREP TIME: 10 minutes ▪ **TOTAL TIME:** 25 minutes

4 cups organic vegetable broth

½ cup coconut aminos

2 cups chopped carrots

1½ cups sliced red onions

1½ teaspoons ginger paste

2 15-ounce cans garbanzo beans, drained and rinsed

3 oranges, peeled and halved

Peel of ¼ orange

⅛ teaspoon ground cinnamon

Pinch of ground nutmeg

Pinch of ground coriander

Sea salt and black pepper to taste

6 slices sprouted-grain bread, toasted

6 cups any Phase 1 fruit

1. Heat a nonstick skillet over medium heat. Put ½ cup of the broth and the coconut aminos in the skillet and heat slightly. Add the carrots, onions, and ginger paste and cook, stirring, for about 10 minutes or until the carrots and onions are soft. Transfer to a mixing bowl. Add the remaining broth, beans, oranges, orange peel, cinnamon, nutmeg, coriander, and salt and pepper.

2. Purée in a blender in batches until smooth. Transfer the soup to a large pot and heat gently. Serve the soup hot, with a slice of toast and 1 cup fruit per serving.

✗

Warm Steak Salad over a Bed of Spinach SERVES 1

PREP TIME: 15 minutes ■ **TOTAL TIME:** 20 minutes

4 ounces New York strip steak, cubed

½ cup diced zucchini or yellow squash

¼ cup sliced red onion

Juice of ½ lime (1 tablespoon)

⅛ teaspoon crushed red pepper flakes

⅛ teaspoon sea salt

⅛ teaspoon chopped fresh cilantro

1 tablespoon organic vegetable broth

½ cup cooked quinoa

½ cup cooked brown or wild rice

2 cups raw spinach

1 cup diced mango

Any Phase 1 dressing

Heat a medium skillet over medium heat and when hot, sauté the steak, squash, onion, lime juice, red pepper flakes, salt, cilantro, and broth and cook, stirring occasionally, until the steak reaches the desired degree of doneness. Mix in the quinoa and rice and serve over a bed of spinach. Garnish with the mango and dress with any Phase 1 dressing.

Hawaiian Burgers SERVES 4

PREP TIME: 10 minutes ■ **TOTAL TIME:** 20 minutes

1 pound lean ground beef

1 cup sprouted-grain bread crumbs

3 garlic cloves

½ cup sliced yellow onion

2 teaspoons sea salt

½ teaspoon black pepper

2 large egg whites or ⅓ cup liquid egg whites

4 thick slices fresh pineapple

1 teaspoon ground cinnamon

¼ cup brown rice, cooked

Mixed greens or spinach

1. Mix together the beef and bread crumbs in a large mixing bowl. Put the garlic and onion in a blender or food processor and purée and when smooth, mix with the beef. Add 1½ teaspoons of the salt, the pepper, and the egg whites and mix well. Divide the mixture and form into four equal-sized patties.

2. Arrange the pineapple slices in a single layer on a plate and sprinkle with the cinnamon and the remaining ½ teaspoon salt.

3. For a stovetop grill pan: Heat the grill pan over medium-high heat and when hot, cook the burgers for about 4 minutes on each side. Cook the pineapple rings at the same time but remove them if they start to char.

4. For an outdoor grill: Heat the grill to about 400°F. Once it is hot, grill the burgers and the pineapple rings for about 4 minutes on each side. If the pineapple rings start to char, remove them before the burgers are done.

5. Top the burgers with the cooked rice and serve with mixed greens or spinach.

TIP: This is incredible for a summer barbeque but notice there is a smaller portion of rice because the burger has bread crumbs in it.

Chicken Sausage Bowl SERVES 3

PREP TIME: 10 minutes ▪ **TOTAL TIME:** 25 minutes

---

4 chicken sausages (or
1 12-ounce pack), diced

½ cup sliced mushrooms

¼ cup sliced red onion

1 red bell pepper, seeded and
sliced

1 green bell pepper, seeded and
sliced

1 teaspoon minced garlic

2 tablespoons organic vegetable
broth

1 sweet potato, baked and diced

1 tablespoon chopped fresh
cilantro

3 cups cooked brown rice

¼ cup salsa

Heat a large nonstick pan over medium heat. Add the sausage and
cook until browned, stirring often. Add the mushrooms, onion, bell
peppers, garlic, and broth and simmer for 3 minutes. Add the sweet
potato and cilantro and cook, stirring often, for about 3 minutes, until the
sweet potato is warm. Pour the mixture over the brown rice and top with
salsa.

Tostada SERVES 1

PREP TIME: 5 minutes ■ **TOTAL TIME:** 5 minutes

½ cup canned black beans, drained and rinsed

¼ cup diced red onion

⅛ teaspoon crushed red pepper flakes

2 tablespoons organic vegetable broth

1 sprouted-grain tortilla, toasted

½ cup arugula

¼ cup sliced jicama

¼ cup chopped tomato

1 tablespoon chopped fresh cilantro

Heat the black beans, onion, red pepper flakes, and broth in a pan over medium heat. When hot, spread the bean mixture down the center of the tortilla. Top with the arugula, jicama, tomato, and cilantro and eat right away.

Sweet Potato Shepherd's Pie SERVES 4

PREP TIME: 10 minutes ■ **TOTAL TIME:** 1 hour 40 minutes

1 cup dry lentils

3 large or 4 medium sweet potatoes, peeled and chopped into ¾-inch cubes

5 carrots, peeled and chopped

2 large onions, chopped

2 garlic cloves, minced

¼ cup organic vegetable broth

2 cups fresh green beans, trimmed and cut into 1-inch pieces

2 teaspoons tamari

1 teaspoon dried thyme

½ teaspoon sea salt

¼ teaspoon black pepper

½ cup unsweetened rice milk

1. Preheat oven to 400°F.

2. In a medium saucepan, combine the lentils with 2 cups of water. Bring to a boil over high heat and immediately reduce the heat and simmer on low for 15 minutes. When cooked, remove from the heat and cover to keep warm.

3. Meanwhile, bring 4 quarts of water to a boil in a large pot. Add the sweet potatoes and boil for 10 minutes, or until tender. Meanwhile, cook the carrots, onions, and garlic in a large skillet with the vegetable broth until the carrots begin to soften. Add the green beans and cook for about 5 minutes more. Add the cooked lentils, tamari, thyme, salt, and pepper. Stir well to combine.

4. Pour the lentil mixture into a large 10-cup casserole dish. Drain and mash the potatoes with the rice milk. Top the lentils with the mashed sweet potatoes and bake for 30 minutes.

TIP: You can adapt this recipe for Phase 3 by sautéing the veggies in 3 or 4 tablespoons of olive oil, and by adding coconut milk to the mashed sweet potatoes. Meat eaters can also substitute 1 pound lean ground beef for the lentils.

Halibut and Veggie Stir-Fry **SERVES 2**

PREP TIME: 10 minutes ▪ **TOTAL TIME:** 20 minutes

1 tablespoon tamari

2 tablespoons coconut aminos

2 tablespoons organic vegetable broth

2 zucchini, sliced

2 yellow squash, sliced

1 red bell pepper, seeded and sliced

1 yellow bell pepper, seeded and sliced

½ cup sliced red onion

1 teaspoon dried cilantro

Juice of ½ lime (1 tablespoon)

2 cups fresh pineapple chunks

12 ounces halibut steak, divided into 2 portions

2 cups cooked brown or wild rice

1. Heat the tamari, 1 tablespoon of the coconut aminos, and 1 tablespoon of the broth in a skillet over medium heat. Add the zucchini, yellow squash, bell peppers, onion, and cilantro and cook for about 15 minutes or until the vegetables are halfway done. Add the lime juice and pineapple, the remaining 1 tablespoon coconut aminos, and the remaining 1 tablespoon broth. Raise the heat to high, add the halibut, and cook to the desired degree of doneness.

2. Serve over a bed of 1 cup rice per serving.

Slow-Cooked Corned Beef and Cabbage SERVES 16

PREP TIME: 10 minutes ▪ **TOTAL TIME:** 7 hours (slow cooker)

5 large carrots, sliced

1 onion, diced

1 cup organic vegetable broth

1 teaspoon fresh or dried thyme

½ teaspoon dry mustard

4 garlic cloves, chopped

1 fresh or dried bay leaf

1 teaspoon peppercorns

4 pounds corned beef brisket

Head of cabbage, coarsely chopped

16 cups cooked brown rice pasta

Put the carrots, onion, broth, thyme, mustard, garlic, bay leaf, pepper-corns, and 4 cups water into a slow cooker or Crock-Pot. Lay the brisket on top and cook on high for 6 hours. Add the cabbage and cook for 1 hour longer or until the cabbage is tender. Remove the bay leaf and serve with the cooked pasta, spooning the juices over the pasta.

Stuffed Cornish Game Hens SERVES 6

PREP TIME: 10 minutes ▪ **TOTAL TIME:** 1 hour 50 minutes

1 cup wild rice

½ cup diced celery

1 red onion, diced

1 green bell pepper, seeded and diced

2 tablespoons tamari

1 teaspoon chopped fresh parsley

½ teaspoon sea salt

3 cups sprouted-grain bread cubes

½ cup organic chicken broth

6 3- to 4-ounce boneless game hen or pheasant breasts

6 slices turkey bacon

¼ teaspoon white pepper

MUSHROOM SAUCE:

¾ cup organic vegetable broth

½ cup sliced mushrooms

½ cup rice milk

¼ cup brown rice flour

¼ cup coconut aminos

1. Rinse the wild rice thoroughly in cold water and put in a medium pot with the celery, onion, bell pepper, tamari, parsley, and salt and ¾ cup of water. Bring to a boil, reduce the heat, and simmer for about 60 minutes or until the rice is tender.

2. Preheat the oven to 375°F.

3. Fold the bread cubes and chicken broth into the rice mixture. In a large baking pan, lay out the game hens and cover with the rice mixture. Lay the turkey bacon across the top of the hens and season with pepper.

4. Stir together the ingredients for the mushroom sauce and pour over the hens. Cover the pan with aluminum foil and bake for about 40 minutes or until the hens are cooked through and the sauce is bubbling hot.

Beef and Cabbage Wraps SERVES 4

PREP TIME: 10 minutes ▦ TOTAL TIME: 30 minutes

1 pound lean ground beef or ground turkey

4 to 6 cups chopped cabbage

½ small white onion, finely chopped

1½ teaspoons sea salt, or to taste

4 spelt, sprouted-grain, or brown rice tortillas

Heat a heavy-bottomed skillet with a lid over medium heat and when hot, cook the ground beef or turkey for about 5 minutes, stirring to break apart, until browned. Add the cabbage and onion and cook, covered, for 20 to 25 minutes, until the veggies are tender. Remove the lid every few minutes to stir. When the cabbage is tender, remove the cover, add the salt and cook for about 5 minutes longer. Warm the tortillas in a separate pan just until soft. Fill the tortillas with the meat mixture and serve warm.

Dover Sole with Tomato and Brown Rice SERVES 6

PREP TIME: 10 minutes ▪ **TOTAL TIME:** 25 minutes

6 cups cooked brown rice

2 tablespoons chopped fresh cilantro

1 tablespoon sea salt herb mix

¼ cup lemon juice

1 tablespoon minced garlic

2 pounds Dover sole or other sole fillets

¼ cup sliced red onion

1 cup chopped tomatoes

1 cup chopped zucchini

1 cup chopped yellow squash

1. Preheat the broiler.

2. Season the rice with 1 tablespoon of the cilantro and 1 teaspoon of the sea salt herb mix and set aside.

3. In a small bowl, combine the lemon juice and garlic, and the remaining 2 teaspoons sea salt herb mix. Lay the fillets on a broiling pan and top with the red onion, tomatoes, zucchini, yellow squash, and the remaining 1 tablespoon of the cilantro. Drizzle the lemon juice mixture over the fish and vegetables. Broil for about 12 minutes or until cooked through. Serve with the rice.

Broccoli and Fava Bean Stir-Fry SERVES 4

PREP TIME: 10 minutes ▪ TOTAL TIME: 25 minutes

1¾ cups organic vegetable broth

1 tablespoon tamari

1 tablespoon tapioca flour

1 tablespoon rice vinegar

1 tablespoon minced ginger

3 tablespoons coconut aminos

4 cups broccoli florets

3 garlic cloves, minced

2 cups cooked fava beans

1 red bell pepper, seeded and cut into thin strips

1½ cups trimmed snow peas

4 green onions (scallions), cut diagonally into ½-inch pieces, white and green parts

4 cups cooked brown or wild rice

1. Mix 1½ cups of the broth with the tamari, tapioca flour, rice vinegar, and ginger in a medium bowl until smooth. Set aside.

2. Heat the coconut aminos in a large, deep skillet or wok over medium-high heat and stir-fry the broccoli and garlic for about 1 minute. Add the remaining ¼ cup of broth, cover, and cook for 5 to 7 minutes, or until the broccoli is tender but still crisp, stirring occasionally. Add the fava beans, bell pepper, snow peas, and green onions and stir-fry for about 3 minutes, until all the vegetables are tender but still crisp.

3. Stir the broth mixture and pour over the vegetables. Bring to a boil over medium heat, stirring constantly. Let the broth boil for 1 minute before ladling equal amounts of the vegetables and broth over the rice.

Pasta and Simmered ✳ Tomato-Meat Sauce SERVES 12

PREP TIME: 15 minutes ■ **TOTAL TIME:** 8 hours (slow cooker)

---

3 pounds lean ground beef

2 cups sliced zucchini

2 cups chopped tomatoes

2 cups cherry tomatoes

2 cups sliced bell peppers

2 cups organic vegetable broth

1 cup sliced onion

1 cup sliced brown mushrooms, such as portobello or shiitake

1 cup sliced light mushrooms, such as button or crimini

½ cup tomato paste

½ cup sliced green onions (scallions), white and green parts

3 tablespoons minced garlic

2 tablespoons sea salt

1 tablespoon chopped fresh parsley

12 cups cooked brown rice pasta

Put all ingredients except the pasta into a slow cooker or Crock-Pot, stir, and cook for 8 hours on low. Spoon equal amounts of the meat sauce over each serving of the pasta and serve.

TIP: Remember, since veggies are unlimited, if you add extra veggies, you can use a larger portion of meat sauce.

Garlic Chicken and Vegetables over Quinoa SERVES 8

PREP TIME: 10 minutes ■ **TOTAL TIME:** 30 minutes

QUINOA:

2 cups quinoa

2 cups organic vegetable broth

2 cups chicken broth

¼ cup sliced onion

¼ cup chopped green onions (scallions), white and green parts

CHICKEN:

2 tablespoons minced garlic

2 pounds boneless, skinless chicken breast, cut into pieces

2 cups sliced bell peppers

2 cups sliced zucchini

2 cups sliced yellow squash

1 cup chopped tomatoes

⅓ cup coconut aminos

1 tablespoon crushed red pepper flakes

1½ teaspoons diced red onion

---

1. In a medium pot, combine the quinoa, vegetable and chicken broths, onion, and green onion. Bring to a boil, reduce the heat, and simmer for 10 to 15 minutes.

2. While the quinoa is cooking, heat a large nonstick skillet over medium heat. Add the garlic and chicken and cook, stirring continuously, until the chicken is browned. Add the bell peppers, zucchini, yellow squash, tomatoes, coconut aminos, red pepper flakes, and red onion. Cook, stirring often, for about 5 minutes, until the vegetables are just tender and the chicken is cooked through.

3. Serve ½ cup of the quinoa topped with 1 cup of the chicken and vegetables.

Ginger Pumpkin-Leek Soup SERVES 3

PREP TIME: 20 minutes ▪ **TOTAL TIME:** 45 minutes

2 medium leeks, halved and thinly sliced

3 garlic cloves, minced

2 cups roasted pumpkin, peeled and seeded, or plain canned pumpkin

1 large sweet potato, cooked, peeled, and cut into chunks

1 medium red bell pepper, seeded and diced

6 cups organic vegetable or chicken broth

1 15-ounce can black beans, drained and rinsed

1 tablespoon tamari

1 tablespoon minced ginger

1 teaspoon ground cumin

2 teaspoons sea salt

4 slices sprouted-grain bread, toasted, or tortillas

¼ cup chopped fresh cilantro (optional)

1. Heat a nonstick skillet over medium heat. Add the leeks and garlic and cook until soft, stirring often. Remove from the heat and set aside.

2. In a large pot, combine the pumpkin, sweet potato, bell pepper, broth, black beans, tamari, ginger, cumin, and salt. Bring to a boil, reduce the heat, and simmer for 15 minutes, stirring occasionally. Add the cooked leeks and combine thoroughly. In a blender, purée the mixture in batches until smooth. Return the soup to the pot and gently heat. Serve hot with a slice of toast or a tortilla and garnish the soup with the cilantro, if using.

Sweet Potato and Broccoli Sauté **SERVES 2**

PREP TIME: 10 minutes ▪ **TOTAL TIME:** 35 minutes

1 large sweet potato, cubed

½ teaspoon coconut aminos, or to taste

½ cup diced yellow onion

2 cups broccoli florets

1 cup canned white beans, rinsed and drained

3 tablespoons tamari

1 tablespoon birch xylitol

1 cup cooked quinoa

1. Put the sweet potato cubes in a pot, cover with water, bring to a boil over medium-high heat. Reduce the heat and simmer briskly for about 15 minutes or until almost tender. Drain the sweet potato and set aside.

2. Heat the coconut aminos in a skillet set over medium-high heat and when hot, sauté the diced onion, broccoli, and beans for 3 or 4 minutes or until they begin to soften. Add the sweet potato and stir to mix.

3. In a bowl, whisk the tamari, xylitol, and 2 tablespoons water until the xylitol is completely dissolved. Pour the xylitol mixture over the vegetables and simmer for about 5 minutes longer or until the vegetables are tender. Serve spooned over the quinoa.

TIP: For meat lovers, swap the white beans for 8 ounces of cubed cooked chicken.

TIP: Because the sweet potatoes are so starchy, I like to serve this dish with just ½ cup of quinoa.

Vegetable Curry SERVES 4 TO 6

PREP TIME: 10 minutes ▮ **TOTAL TIME:** 4 to 8 hours (slow cooker)

4 sweet potatoes, diced

2 large tomatoes, chopped

1 onion, diced

1 red bell pepper, seeded and chopped

1 cup diced carrots

1 cup green beans

1 cup broccoli florets

1 15-ounce can garbanzo beans, drained and rinsed

1 6-ounce can tomato paste

2 teaspoons curry powder

½ teaspoon minced garlic

½ teaspoon sea salt

3 cups cooked brown rice or spelt pasta

Put all ingredients except the pasta into a slow cooker or Crock-Pot with ¾ cup water, stir, and cook for 4 to 6 hours on high or 6 to 8 hours on low. Serve with the pasta.

✳ Vegetarian Lentil Chili SERVES 8

PREP TIME: 10 minutes ▪ **TOTAL TIME:** 3 to 8 hours (slow cooker)

---

1 cup lentils, rinsed

2 cups diced tomatoes

1 15-ounce can black beans, drained and rinsed

1 15-ounce can white or cannellini beans, drained and rinsed

4 cups organic vegetable broth

1½ cups diced red onion

½ cup diced celery

2 garlic cloves, minced

2 tablespoons tamari

2 tablespoons chili powder

1 tablespoon ground cumin

8 cups cooked brown rice or brown rice pasta

Put all ingredients except the rice or pasta into a slow cooker or Crock-Pot and cook for 3 to 4 hours on high or 7 to 8 hours on low. Serve over the rice.

Cinnamon-Dusted Apple SERVES 1

PREP TIME: 2 minutes ■ **TOTAL TIME:** 2 minutes

1 apple   **Ground cinnamon to taste**

Core and slice the apple and sprinkle with cinnamon just before eating.

Papaya with Lime Juice SERVES 1

PREP TIME: 2 minutes ■ **TOTAL TIME:** 2 minutes

Lime juice to taste   **1 cup diced papaya**

Squeeze lime juice over the papaya and enjoy.

Cucumber and Tangerine Salad SERVES 1

PREP TIME: 2 minutes ■ **TOTAL TIME:** 2 minutes

1 cup diced cucumbers

1 tangerine, peeled, segmented, and cut into ½-inch pieces

1 tablespoon rice vinegar

⅛ teaspoon stevia

⅛ teaspoon fresh dill weed

Toss the cucumbers and tangerine with the vinegar, stevia, and dill. Serve immediately.

Chili-Kissed Mangos SERVES 1

PREP TIME: 2 minutes ■ **TOTAL TIME:** 2 minutes

Chili powder to taste

1 cup sliced mango

Sprinkle chili powder on the mango slices and enjoy.

Ginger Peaches **SERVES 1**

PREP TIME: 2 minutes ■ **TOTAL TIME:** 2 minutes

1 cup chopped peaches

¼ teaspoon minced ginger

Top the peaches with the ginger and enjoy.

Grapefruit with Cinnamon **SERVES 1**

PREP TIME: 2 minutes ■ **TOTAL TIME:** 2 minutes

Ground cinnamon to taste
⅛ teaspoon stevia

1 grapefruit

Sprinkle cinnamon and stevia on the grapefruit and serve.

Minty Jicama Fruit Salad SERVES 1

PREP TIME: 5 minutes ■ **TOTAL TIME:** 5 minutes

1 cup of any combination of Phase 1 fruits

½ cup sliced jicama

3 sliced cucumbers

DRESSING:

5 fresh mint leaves, chopped

1 teaspoon birch xylitol

Juice of 2 limes (¼ cup)

Dice the fruit and combine with the jicama and cucumbers. To make the dressing, mix the mint leaves and xylitol with the lime juice. Toss gently with the fruit and serve right away.

TIP: I love to use Persian cucumbers in this recipe

Watermelon with Mint SERVES 1

PREP TIME: 2 minutes ▪ **TOTAL TIME:** 2 minutes

---

1 cup cubed watermelon   **2 fresh mint leaves, chopped**

Top the watermelon cubes with the mint and enjoy.

Spicy Pomegranate Seeds SERVES 1

PREP TIME: 2 minutes ▪ **TOTAL TIME:** 2 minutes

Chili powder to taste   **1 cup pomegranate seeds**

Sprinkle the chili powder on the pomegranate seeds and enjoy.

Quinoa-Pear Smoothie SERVES 1

PREP TIME: 5 minutes ■ **TOTAL TIME:** 5 minutes

¼ cup cooked quinoa

½ cup rice milk

1 pear, cored, seeded, and stemmed

Pinch of ground cinnamon

Pinch of ground nutmeg

1 cup ice cubes

Blend all the ingredients until smooth. Serve immediately.

Three-Melon Smoothie with Mint SERVES 2

PREP TIME: 5 minutes ■ **TOTAL TIME:** 5 minutes

¾ cup diced cantaloupe

¾ cup diced honeydew melon

½ cup diced watermelon

5 fresh mint leaves

Juice of ½ lime (1 tablespoon)

1 cup ice cubes

Blend all the ingredients with ½ cup of cold water until smooth. Serve immediately.

Green Apple Smoothie SERVES 1

PREP TIME: 2 minutes ■ **TOTAL TIME:** 2 minutes

1 cup spinach
1 cup kale

1 green apple, cored and diced

Blend all the ingredients with 1 cup of cold water until smooth. Serve immediately

TIP: Some people like to remove the ribs of the kale because they can be a bit bitter. But I leave them in because they help with digestion. You can always add some birch xylitol, stevia, or a pinch of cinnamon to taste to mask the bitterness.

Tropical Smoothie SERVES 2

PREP TIME: 5 minutes ▪ **TOTAL TIME:** 5 minutes

½ cup diced pineapple
½ cup seeded, diced papaya

1 kiwi, peeled and chopped
1 cup ice cubes

Blend all the ingredients with 1 cup of cold water until smooth. Serve immediately

Cantaloupe Smoothie SERVES 1

PREP TIME: 2 minutes ▪ **TOTAL TIME:** 2 minutes

1 cup diced cantaloupe
1 fresh mint leaf

2 cups ice cubes

Blend all the ingredients with ½ cup cold water until smooth. Serve immediately

One serving for all dips and dressings is 2 to 4 tablespoons.

Black Bean Cilantro Dip SERVES 1

PREP TIME: 2 minutes ■ **TOTAL TIME:** 2 minutes

2 tablespoons cooked or canned black beans

1 tablespoon tamari

1 tablespoon organic vegetable broth

¼ teaspoon chopped fresh cilantro

Blend all the ingredients until smooth. Serve as a dip with any Phase 1 veggies.

TIP: My clients like to make big batches of these dressings and freeze them in single serving ziplock bags and label them Phase 1 dressing. Just take a Phase 1 dinner, put the leftovers on a bed of lettuce, grab a bag of dressing and a fruit and you're ready to brown bag it for lunch.

Tangerine-Cucumber Dressing SERVES 3

PREP TIME: 2 minutes ▪ TOTAL TIME: 2 minutes

1 tangerine, peeled and seeded

½ cup diced cucumber

2 tablespoons water

Pinch of stevia

⅛ teaspoon chopped fresh parsley

Sea salt and white pepper to taste

Blend all the ingredients with 2 tablespoons water until smooth. Serve as a dip or drizzled over any dish that needs a dressing.

White Bean-Dill Dip SERVES 6 TO 8

PREP TIME: 2 minutes ▪ TOTAL TIME: 2 minutes

1 15-ounce can white beans, drained

½ teaspoon chopped fresh dill weed

¼ cup tamari

Blend the ingredients with ¼ cup water until smooth. Serve as a dip with any Phase 1 veggies.

Chunky Mango Salsa SERVES 2

PREP TIME: 5 minutes ■ TOTAL TIME: 5 minutes

½ cup diced mango

¼ cup diced tomato

¼ cup diced red onion

¼ tablespoon chopped fresh cilantro

Stir all ingredients in a small bowl to serve as a dip or blend all ingredients until smooth to drizzle as a dressing.

Herbed White Bean Spread SERVES 6 TO 8

PREP TIME: 5 minutes ■ TOTAL TIME: 5 minutes

1 15-ounce can garbanzo beans, drained and rinsed

Juice of 1 lemon (3 tablespoons)

2 garlic cloves

2 tablespoons coconut aminos

1 teaspoon chopped fresh parsley

⅛ teaspoon fresh dill weed

⅛ teaspoon sea salt

⅛ teaspoon white pepper

Blend the ingredients to the desired consistency. Add warm water as needed to thin the spread. Serve as a dip.

Quick Baked Apple Crisp SERVES 1

PREP TIME: 5 minutes ▪ TOTAL TIME: 25 minutes

1 apple, cored and diced into ½-inch cubes

1 teaspoon tapioca flour

1 teaspoon rice milk

⅛ teaspoon ground cinnamon

Pinch of ground nutmeg

Pinch of stevia

1. Preheat the oven to 400°F.

2. Mix the ingredients in an oven-safe baking dish and bake for 15 to 20 minutes. Serve the crisp hot, warm, or chilled.

TIP: Remember, because this dessert contains fruit, you cannot eat it with a Phase 1 dinner. Feel free to enjoy it as a snack, or add it to your lunch as long as you also add another day of phase-specific exercise.

Mint Grilled Pineapple SERVES 1

PREP TIME: 5 minutes ▪ TOTAL TIME: 5 minutes

1 cup sliced fresh pineapple   2 fresh mint leaves, chopped

Broil or grill the pineapple slices for 2 to 3 minutes on each side until softened and lightly browned. Sprinkle with the mint leaves and serve.

TIP: You can eat this yummy dessert as a Phase 1 snack.

Strawberry-Beet Sorbet SERVES 2

PREP TIME: 2 minutes ▪ TOTAL TIME: 2 minutes

2 cups strawberries, stemmed   ¼ cup birch xylitol
¼ cup diced beets   4 cups ice cubes

Blend the ingredients until smooth. Serve right away.

Orange Sorbet SERVES 2

PREP TIME: 2 minutes ■ **TOTAL TIME:** 2 minutes

2 cups peeled orange segments

2 tablespoons birch xylitol

4 cups ice cubes

Blend the ingredients until smooth. Serve right away.

TIP: For peach sorbet, substitute an equal amount of peaches for the oranges.

Pumpkin Cookies SERVES 1

PREP TIME: 10 minutes ■ **TOTAL TIME:** 1 hour (plus cooling time)

3 large room-temperature egg whites

⅛ teaspoon cream of tartar

¼ teaspoon vanilla extract

½ teaspoon lemon juice

½ cup birch xylitol

¼ cup pumpkin purée

½ teaspoon cinnamon

pinch of nutmeg, ginger, and allspice

1. Preheat oven to 300°F. Line a baking sheet with parchment paper. Beat the egg whites on low-medium speed until foamy. Add the cream of tartar, vanilla, and lemon juice, and continue beating until soft peaks form. Add the xylitol gradually. Beat until stiff peaks form.

2. In a bowl, mix the purée with the spices. Carefully fold in ¼ of the meringue. Gently fold the pumpkin mixture back into the meringue. Drop mounds of meringue onto the prepared sheet. Bake about 50 minutes until fairly crisp. Allow cookies to dry for several hours.

TIP: Because these do not contain fruit they can't be swapped for a snack, but enjoy them with a phase 1 lunch or dinner (just add your day of exercise).

Phase 1 Food List

To modify any of the recipes for this phase of the diet, or to make up your own, you may use any of the foods on the following Phase 1 food list.

VEGETABLES AND SALAD GREENS (fresh, canned, or frozen)

Arrowroot

Arugula

Bamboo shoots

Beans: *green, yellow (wax), French*

Beets

Broccoli florets

Cabbage, all types

Carrots

Celery, including tops

Cucumbers

Eggplant

Green chiles

Green onions

Jicama

Kale

Leeks

Lettuce (any except iceberg)

Mixed greens

Mushrooms

Onions, red and yellow

Parsnips

Peas: *snap, snow*

Peppers: *bell, pepperoncini*

Pumpkin

Radishes

Rutabaga

Spinach

Spirulina

Sprouts

Sweet potatoes/ yams

Tomatoes

Turnips

Zucchini and winter or yellow summer squash

FRUITS (fresh or frozen)

Apples

Apricots

Asian pears

Berries: *blackberries. blueberries, mulberries, raspberries*

Cantaloupe

Cherries

Figs

Grapefruit

Guava

Honeydew melon

Kiwis

Kumquats

Lemons

Limes

Loganberries

Mangos

Oranges

Papaya

Peaches

Pears

Pineapples

Pomegranates

Strawberries

Tangerines

Watermelon

ANIMAL PROTEIN

Beef: *filet, lean ground*

Buffalo meat, ground

Chicken: *boneless, skinless white meat*

Corned beef

Deli meats, nitrate-free: *turkey, chicken, roast beef*

Eggs, whites only

Game: *partridge, pheasant*

Guinea fowl

Haddock fillet

Halibut: *fillet, steak*

Pollock fillet

Pork: *tenderloin*

Sardines, packed in water

Sausages, nitrate-free: *turkey, chicken*

Sole fillet

Tuna, fresh or solid white, packed in water

Turkey: *breast meat, lean ground*

Turkey bacon: *nitrate-free*

VEGETABLE PROTEIN

Black-eyed peas

Chana dal/lentils

Chickpeas/
garbanzo beans

Dried or canned
beans: *adzuki,
black, butter, great
northern, kidney,*

*lima, navy, pinto,
white*

Fava beans, fresh
or canned

BROTHS, HERBS, SPICES, CONDIMENTS, AND SUPPLEMENTS

Brewer's yeast

Broths: *beef,
chicken, vegetable**

Dried herbs: *all
types*

Fresh herbs: *all
types*

Garlic, fresh

Ginger, fresh

Horseradish,
prepared

Ketchup, no sugar
added, no corn
syrup

Mustard,
prepared, dry

Natural
seasonings: *Bragg
Liquid Aminos,
coconut amino
acids, tamari*

Noncaffeinated
herbal teas or
Pero

Nutritional yeast

Pickles, no sugar
added

Salsa

Seasonings: *black
and white peppers,
cinnamon, chili
powder, crushed
red pepper flakes,
cumin, curry
powder, nutmeg,
onion salt, raw
cacao powder,*

*turmeric, sea salt,
Simply Organic
seasoning*

Sweeteners:
*stevia, xylitol (birch
only)*

Tomato paste

Tomato soup

Vanilla or
peppermint
extract

Vinegar: *any type*

GRAINS AND STARCHES

Amaranth

Arrowroot

Barley

Brown rice: *rice,
cereal, crackers,
flour, pasta, tortillas*

Brown rice cheese
or milk

Buckwheat

Gluten-free
pancake mix

Kamut

Millet

Oats: *steel-cut,
old-fashioned*

Quinoa

Rice milk, plain

Spelt: *pasta,
pretzels, tortillas*

Sprouted-grain:
*bagels, bread,
tortillas*

Tapioca

Teff

Triticale

Wild rice

HEALTHY FATS

None for this
phase

*NOTE: All broths, if possible, should be free of additives and preservatives.

PHASE 2

Breakfast
Smoked Salmon and Cucumber
Jicama with Bacon and Lime
Bacon-Wrapped Asparagus
Spinach and Mushroom Scramble
Hard-Boiled Egg Whites Stuffed with Minced Veggies
Rhubarb Meringue
Steak and Eggs
Pork and Collard Greens
Southwestern Breakfast Stir-Fry
Tempeh-Mushroom Hash (vegans only)
Egg White and Broccoli Omelet

Lunch
Mustardy Roast Beef Lettuce Wrap
Tuna Salad in Endive Leaves
Edamame Chopped Confetti Salad (vegans only)
Buffalo Tip Salad
Chicken Fajita Salad
Home-style Turkey Meat Loaf
Green Beans and Ground Turkey in Butter Lettuce Cups
Lemon-Broiled Chicken
Lemon-Pepper Filet Mignon and Cabbage
Broiled Mustard-Coated Steak
Buffalo Wrap
Lemon-Dressed Tuna Salad
Warm Asparagus and Bacon Salad

Dinner
Chicken with Shiitake Mushrooms and Mustard Greens
Marinated Chicken and Veggie Kabobs
Long and Slow Beef Stew
Turkey Meat Loaf and Asparagus
Baked Cod and Veggies
Steak Fajita Lettuce Wraps
Rosemary Pork Tenderloin with Mustard Greens
Sardine Salad with Kale and Bacon
Lemon Mustard Pepper Chicken

Greek Meatballs and Veggies
New York Strip Steak with Broccoli
Edamame and Leek Salad (vegans only)
Tempeh Vegetable Stew (vegans only)
Portobello Mushrooms and Mustard Greens
Garden Egg White Scramble
Three-Pepper Egg White Soufflé

Snacks
Mustard Egg Salad
Roast Beef–Wrapped Pickles
Smoked Salmon and Celery
Wild Sardine Pâté
Red Pepper Stuffed with Crunchy Tuna Salad
Garden Meatballs
Summer Salsa with Turkey Bacon Chips
Leftover Lettuce Cups with Dressing
Oysters on Cucumbers
Salty Edamame (vegans only)
Sardine and Cucumber Canapés
Peppery Tofu Jerky (vegans only)

Smoothies/Beverages
Arnold Palmer
Lime-Mint Smoothie
Homemade Lemonade
Colon Cleanse Smoothie
Detox Smoothie
Sun Tea Mojito

Dips and Dressings
Red Bell Pepper Dressing
Pepperoncini Dressing
Lemon Vinaigrette
Chipotle Dressing
Fiery Southwestern Dip

Desserts
Lime Sorbet
Lemon Meringue
Lemon and Lime Ice Pops

Smoked Salmon and Cucumber **SERVES 1**

PREP TIME: 2 minutes ■ **TOTAL TIME:** 2 minutes

1 cucumber

6 ounces smoked salmon,
nitrate-free, no sugar added

¼ teaspoon lime juice (optional)

Pinch of fresh dill weed
(optional)

Slice the cucumber into rounds, approximately ½ inch thick. Slice the salmon into 1-inch pieces. Put the salmon pieces on the cucumber rounds. Drizzle with lime juice or season with dill weed, if using.

TIP: Feel free to use extra cucumber with the hearty amount of salmon. Remember, veggies are unlimited!

Jicama with Bacon and Lime **SERVES 1**

PREP TIME: 5 minutes ■ **TOTAL TIME:** 5 minutes

4 slices turkey bacon
½ cup diced jicama

Juice of ¼ lime (1½ teaspoons)

Cook the turkey bacon according to the package directions, drain, slice, and transfer to a mixing bowl. Add the jicama and lime juice. Stir and serve.

Bacon-Wrapped Asparagus SERVES 1

PREP TIME: 5 minutes ■ **TOTAL TIME:** 25 minutes

4 asparagus spears

4 slices turkey bacon

2 tablespoons organic vegetable broth

1. Preheat the oven to 375°F.

2. Rinse the asparagus spears and snap or cut off the tough stems. Wrap a slice of turkey bacon around each spear and lay them on a rimmed baking sheet. Add the broth, cover with aluminum foil and bake for about 20 minutes or until the asparagus is tender and the bacon cooked.

Spinach and Mushroom Scramble SERVES 1

PREP TIME: 5 minutes ▪ **TOTAL TIME:** 10 minutes

4 slices turkey bacon, diced

½ cup sliced mushrooms

½ cup chopped spinach

¼ cup diced onion

2 tablespoons organic vegetable broth

Sea salt and black pepper to taste

Heat a large skillet over medium heat and when hot, cook the ingredients for about 5 minutes, until the onion is soft and the bacon cooked. Serve immediately.

TIP: I love this meal so much that I've been known to double the portion, have one for breakfast, and split the second over two Phase 2 snacks (because remember, your portion for protein is half the size for snacks).

VEGGIE SWAP (VEGANS ONLY): Substitute 4 ounces extra-firm tofu, cut into bite-size chunks, for the turkey bacon. Brown the tofu in a dry nonstick skillet over medium heat. Add all other ingredients and sauté until the onion is translucent.

Hard-Boiled Egg Whites Stuffed with Minced Veggies *

SERVES 1

PREP TIME: 2 minutes ▪ **TOTAL TIME:** 2 minutes

3 large hard-boiled eggs	½ cup cooked, minced Phase 2 veggies

Peel the eggs, cut them in half lengthwise, and discard the yolks. Fill with the minced veggies and serve right away.

TIP: When I make this recipe, I often use my leftover vegetables from the night before. Try it with onions, mushrooms, bell peppers, or cabbage.

Rhubarb Meringue SERVES 3

PREP TIME: 10 minutes ■ **TOTAL TIME:** 30 minutes

3 cups chopped rhubarb

¾ cup birch xylitol

½ teaspoon ground cinnamon

3 tablespoons arrowroot powder

1 teaspoon vanilla extract

6 large egg whites or 1 cup liquid egg whites

2 tablespoons chopped lemon zest

1. Preheat the oven to 350°F.

2. In a saucepan set over medium heat, bring the rhubarb, ½ cup of the xylitol, cinnamon, and 5 tablespoons of water to a boil and cook for about 10 minutes or until the rhubarb is tender. Reduce the heat to a simmer, add the arrowroot and vanilla and continue cooking, stirring often, until the sauce thickens.

3. In a clean glass bowl, whisk the egg whites until soft peaks form. Gradually add the remaining ¼ cup xylitol and continue whisking until stiff peaks form.

4. Spoon ½ cup of the rhubarb into each of three individual, oven-safe custard cups. Top each cup with equal amounts of the meringue and sprinkle with lemon zest. Bake for 10 minutes, or until the meringue is light golden brown.

Steak and Eggs SERVES 1 ✳

PREP TIME: 5 minutes ■ **TOTAL TIME:** 15 minutes

- 2 ounces sirloin steak, sliced
- ¼ cup sliced red onion
- ¼ cup diced bell pepper
- 1 tablespoon coconut aminos

- 2 large egg whites or ⅓ cup liquid egg whites
- Sea salt and black pepper to taste

Heat a medium skillet over medium heat and cook the steak, onion, bell pepper, and coconut aminos for 3 to 5 minutes or until the steak reaches the desired degree of doneness. Add the egg whites and cook, stirring, for about 5 minutes or until they become firm. Season with salt and pepper.

TIP: I often use leftover steak from the night before. This makes a super quick breakfast. You can also replace the sirloin steak with lean ground beef or London broil.

Pork and Collard Greens SERVES 1

PREP TIME: 2 minutes ▪ **TOTAL TIME:** 15 minutes

4 ounces pork tenderloin, diced

1 tablespoon tamari

¼ teaspoon crushed red pepper flakes

¼ teaspoon dry mustard

¼ teaspoon minced garlic

¼ teaspoon sea salt

¼ teaspoon black pepper

1 cup collard greens, stemmed and sliced into ½-inch strips

Heat a skillet over medium heat and cook the pork, tamari, red pepper flakes, mustard, garlic, salt, and pepper, stirring occasionally, for 8 to 10 minutes or until the pork is fully cooked. Add the collard greens and cook for about 5 minutes, until the greens soften and wilt.

Southwestern Breakfast Stir-Fry SERVES 1

PREP TIME: 5 minutes ▪ **TOTAL TIME:** 15 minutes

- 4 ounces lean ground beef
- ½ cup diced cabbage
- ¼ cup chopped Hatch green chile
- ¼ cup chopped onion
- ½ teaspoon crushed red pepper flakes
- ½ teaspoon chopped fresh cilantro
- ½ bell pepper, top cut off, seeded
- ½ teaspoon lime juice

Heat a medium nonstick skillet over medium heat and when hot, cook the beef, cabbage, chile, onion, red pepper flakes, and cilantro, stirring often, for about 7 minutes or until the beef is cooked. Stuff the bell pepper with the beef mixture and drizzle with the lime juice.

VEGAN SWAP: Substitute 4 ounces diced tempeh for the ground beef and cook as directed. Remember, because tempeh contains soy, this is an exception for my vegan friends.

Tempeh-Mushroom Hash SERVES 2

PREP TIME: 10 minutes ■ **TOTAL TIME:** 30 minutes

- 8 ounces tempeh, cut into small cubes
- 1 cup diced onion
- ½ cup diced red bell pepper
- 2½ cups sliced mushrooms (baby portobello or other variety)
- 1 tablespoon balsamic vinegar
- 5 cups baby spinach
- Black pepper, to taste
- Pinch of ground nutmeg

Heat a large nonstick skillet over medium-high heat and when hot, cook tempeh until browned, stirring often, about 5 minutes. Push the tempeh to the side of the pan, add the onion and bell pepper, and sauté for about 5 minutes. Add the mushrooms and cook, stirring often, for about 5 minutes more, until browned. Add the balsamic vinegar, reduce the heat, and cover the pan, and cook for about 3 minutes. Add the spinach and cook for an additional 2 minutes just until the spinach is heated through and starts to soften. Season with the pepper and nutmeg.

TIP: Keeps well, so store the rest for tomorrow's breakfast or lunch!

NOTE: Because it contains tempeh, this recipe is only for vegans or vegetarians who do not eat eggs.

Egg White and Broccoli Omelet SERVES 1

PREP TIME: 5 minutes ▪ **TOTAL TIME:** 25 minutes

1 tablespoon chopped onion

1 tablespoon chopped shallot

1 tablespoon minced garlic

½ cup chopped fresh broccoli

3 large egg whites or ½ cup liquid egg whites

Pinch of sea salt

Cook the onion, shallot, and garlic in a nonstick skillet over medium-high heat for 5 to 6 minutes or until soft. Stir in the broccoli and cook for about 10 minutes longer or until soft. Mix in the egg whites and stir to scramble. Let the eggs cook to the desired consistency. Sprinkle with salt and serve.

Mustardy Roast Beef Lettuce Wrap **SERVES 1**

PREP TIME: 2 minutes ▪ **TOTAL TIME:** 2 minutes

4 ounces nitrate-free sliced roast beef

Lettuce leaves

1 tablespoon Dijon mustard

5 to 6 red onion slices

Arrange the slices of beef in the lettuce leaves (you probably will use 2 leaves) and spread the mustard over the meat. Scatter the onions over the beef and gently fold the lettuce around the filling to cup it. Eat immediately.

TIP: I love this with turkey and pickles too!

Tuna Salad in Endive Leaves SERVES 1

PREP TIME: 5 minutes ■ **TOTAL TIME:** 5 minutes

6 ounces water-packed tuna, drained

¼ cup fresh watercress

¼ cup diced dill pickle, no preservatives, no sugars added

2 tablespoons diced red onion

1 tablespoon coconut vinegar

Sea salt and black pepper to taste

4 endive leaves

In a small bowl, mix together the tuna, watercress, pickles, onion, and vinegar. Season with salt and pepper. Scoop the tuna salad into the endive leaves so that they cup the filling. Eat immediately.

VEGGIE SWAP: Substitute ½ cup edamame for the tuna. Cook frozen edamame in the microwave with a small amount of water in a covered dish for 2 to 3 minutes. Drain and rinse with cold water.

TIP: Many of my clients have severe food allergies and coconut vinegar is one of the few vinegars many of them can tolerate. Plus, it tastes good! You can find it at your local health food store or order it online.

Edamame Chopped Confetti Salad SERVES 1

PREP TIME: 5 minutes ▪ **TOTAL TIME:** 5 minutes

½ cup edamame, cooked and cooled

½ cup chopped broccoli

½ cup diced red bell pepper

¼ cup diced cucumber

¼ cup diced green onion (scallion), white and green parts

¼ cup diced pepperoncini

Lime juice to taste

Tamari to taste

In a medium bowl, toss edamame and broccoli with the bell pepper, cucumber, green onion, and pepperoncini. Dress with lime juice and a splash of tamari.

NOTE: Because it contains edamame (soy beans), this recipe is only for vegans or vegetarians who do not eat eggs.

Buffalo Tip Salad SERVES 1

PREP TIME: 5 minutes ■ **TOTAL TIME:** 15 minutes

4 ounces buffalo tri-tips, sliced into 2 × ½-inch strips

Juice of ½ lime (1 tablespoon)

⅛ teaspoon crushed red pepper flakes

⅛ teaspoon chili powder

Pinch of sea salt

2 to 4 cups mixed greens

½ cup diced cucumber

¼ cup sliced green onion (scallion), white and green parts

Any Phase 2 dressing

1. Preheat the broiler.

2. Dress the buffalo strips with the lime juice, red pepper flakes, chili powder, and salt. Lay the strips on a broiling pan and broil for 5 to 7 minutes or to the desired degree of doneness. Serve over a bed of mixed greens tossed with cucumber and green onion and dressed with any Phase 2 dressing.

Chicken Fajita Salad SERVES 4

PREP TIME: 10 minutes ■ **TOTAL TIME:** 25 minutes

¼ cup coconut aminos

4 small boneless, skinless chicken breasts (about 1 pound), cut into bite-size pieces

1 bell pepper, seeded and cut into long julienne strips

1 medium white onion, cut into rounds

¼ to ½ teaspoon mild chili powder, or to taste

¼ teaspoon sea salt, or to taste

4 cups torn lettuce

Put 2 tablespoons of the coconut aminos in a large nonstick skillet over medium heat and when hot, cook the chicken for about 7 minutes or until lightly browned. Add the bell pepper, onion, chili powder, salt, and the remaining 2 tablespoons coconut aminos. Cook for about 5 minutes more, until the onion is soft. Serve over lettuce.

Home-style Turkey Meat Loaf SERVES 8

PREP TIME: 5 minutes ▪ **TOTAL TIME:** 1 hour 15 minutes

2 pounds ground turkey

2 large egg whites or ⅓ cup liquid egg whites

2 tablespoons coconut aminos

½ cup diced onion

½ cup chopped celery

1 teaspoon minced garlic

1 teaspoon sea salt

1 teaspoon black pepper

4 to 6 cups steamed broccoli

1. Preheat the oven to 375°F.

2. Combine the turkey, egg whites, coconut aminos, onion, celery, garlic, salt, and pepper in a large mixing bowl. When well mixed, press the mixture into a nonstick loaf pan and bake for about 1 hour or until cooked through. Let rest for 10 minutes. Slice and serve with steamed broccoli.

Green Beans and Ground Turkey in Butter Lettuce Cups SERVES 4

PREP TIME: 10 minutes ■ **TOTAL TIME:** 25 minutes

1 pound lean ground turkey

3 cups chopped green beans

½ cup diced red onions

3 tablespoons coconut aminos

3 tablespoons organic vegetable broth

¼ teaspoon fresh ground pepper

⅛ teaspoon sea salt

4 butter lettuce leaves

½ cup any Phase 2 dressing

1. In a large nonstick skillet, cook the turkey, stirring to break up the meat, for 2 to 3 minutes. Add the beans, onions, aminos, and broth, season with pepper and salt and continue to cook, stirring frequently, for 10 to 12 minutes or until the turkey is cooked through and the beans are fork tender.

2. Spoon the mixture into the lettuce leaf cups and drizzle with equal amounts of dressing.

Lemon-Broiled ✗ Chicken SERVES 4

PREP TIME: 5 minutes ▪ **TOTAL TIME:** 2 to 4 hours (includes marinating time)

2 tablespoons finely chopped fresh basil

2 tablespoons organic vegetable broth

2 tablespoons spicy mustard

Juice of 1 lemon (3 tablespoons)

Dash of sea salt

Dash of black pepper

4 small boneless, skinless chicken breasts (about 1 pound)

1. In a small bowl, stir together the basil, broth, mustard, lemon juice, salt, and pepper. Transfer to a gallon-size food storage bag and add the chicken. Close the bag and shake it to coat the chicken with the marinade. Make sure the bag is tightly sealed and refrigerate for 2 to 4 hours.

2. Preheat the grill or broiler.

3. Remove the chicken from the bag and let any excess marinade drip from the pieces. Discard the marinade. Grill or broil the chicken for 5 to 7 minutes on each side, until it is cooked through.

Lemon-Pepper Filet Mignon and Cabbage SERVES 1

PREP TIME: 5 minutes ■ **TOTAL TIME:** 15 minutes

4 ounces filet mignon

2 teaspoons cider vinegar

½ teaspoon lemon pepper

⅛ teaspoon finely chopped fresh rosemary leaves

1 cup shredded cabbage

Pinch of stevia

1. Season the filet with 1 teaspoon of the vinegar, ¼ teaspoon of the lemon pepper, and the rosemary. Gently rub the seasonings into the meat. Heat a heavy-bottomed pan over medium heat and sauté the filet for 2 to 3 minutes on each side or cooked to the desired degree of doneness. Let the filet rest for 5 minutes and then slice it very thin.

2. Put the cabbage, stevia, 1 tablespoon of water, the remaining teaspoon of vinegar, and remaining ¼ teaspoon of lemon pepper in a small saucepan. Cook the cabbage over medium heat, stirring often, for 3 to 5 minutes, or until barely tender. Take care not to overcook the cabbage; it should be crispy. Serve the sliced filet over a bed of cabbage.

Broiled Mustard-Coated Steak SERVES 1

PREP TIME: 15 minutes ▪ **TOTAL TIME:** 30 minutes

2 teaspoons balsamic vinegar

2 garlic cloves, minced

1 teaspoon dry mustard

½ teaspoon black pepper

¼ teaspoon sea salt

4 ounces sirloin steak or flank steak (like London broil)

Mixed greens

Any Phase 2 dressing

1. Preheat the broiler.

2. Line a broiling pan with aluminum foil.

3. In a bowl, mix together the vinegar, garlic, mustard, pepper, and salt. Put the steak on the prepared pan and spread the mustard mixture over it. Let the steak stand for about 10 minutes to give the flavors time to develop. Broil the steak for 3 to 4 minutes on each side for medium-rare, or until it reaches the desired degree of doneness. Let the beef rest for 5 minutes before slicing and serving over a bed of mixed greens drizzled with a Phase 2 dressing.

Buffalo Wrap SERVES 4

PREP TIME: 10 minutes ■ **TOTAL TIME:** 25 minutes

8 large cabbage leaves

1 teaspoon coconut aminos

1 small onion, chopped

1 tablespoon chopped garlic

1 sprig fresh rosemary, stemmed and chopped

1 pound ground buffalo or bison

1. Put the cabbage leaves in a large pot and fill it with water. Bring the water to a boil over medium-high heat, and immediately reduce the heat to a simmer. Simmer briskly for about 2 minutes, or until the cabbage is just tender. Do not overcook. Lift the leaves from the water and drain on paper towels.

2. Heat a heavy-bottomed skillet over medium heat and when hot, cook the coconut aminos, onion, garlic, and rosemary for about 5 minutes or until the onion is translucent. Remove the onions from the pan and set aside. Reheat the pan over medium heat and when hot, cook the buffalo, stirring often to break up the meat, for about 5 minutes or until browned. Return the onions to the pan, stir, and remove from the heat. On a plate or flat surface, position a cabbage leaf with the stem side away from you. Spoon an eighth of the meat filling into the leaf, fold in the sides of the leaf, and gently roll. Put the roll, seam side down, on a serving plate and repeat with the remaining 7 cabbage leaves. Serve immediately.

Lemon-Dressed ✶ Tuna Salad SERVES 1

PREP TIME: 5 minutes ■ **TOTAL TIME:** 1 hour 5 minutes

6 ounces water-packed tuna, drained

¼ cup shredded red cabbage

½ cup diced cucumber

2 teaspoons minced red onion

1 tablespoon vinegar

1 tablespoon lemon juice

Pinch of stevia

Pinch of fresh dill weed

Put the tuna, cabbage, cucumber, and onion in a medium bowl. In another small bowl, stir together the vinegar, lemon juice, stevia, and dill weed. Toss the tuna mixture with the vinegar mixture and refrigerate for at least 1 hour.

TIP: You can stuff this in endive or a bell pepper.

✻ Warm Asparagus and Bacon Salad SERVES 1

PREP TIME: 5 minutes ■ **TOTAL TIME:** 10 minutes

6 asparagus spears

4 slices turkey bacon

2 tablespoons diced red onion

1 tablespoon organic vegetable broth

Snap or cut off the tough lower stems from the asparagus spears and discard. Cut the remaining spears into 1-inch lengths. Cut the turkey bacon into 1-inch lengths. Heat a skillet over medium heat and when hot, sauté the asparagus, bacon, onion and broth for about 8 minutes or until the asparagus is soft.

Chicken with Shiitake Mushrooms and Mustard Greens **SERVES 4**

PREP TIME: 5 minutes ■ **TOTAL TIME:** 25 minutes

- 1 pound boneless, skinless chicken breast, diced into 1-inch cubes
- ¼ cup organic vegetable broth
- Bunch of mustard greens, roughly chopped
- 2 cups shiitake mushrooms, stemmed and chopped
- 4 garlic cloves, minced
- 1 tablespoon minced ginger
- 1 tablespoon coconut vinegar
- Bunch of green onions (scallions), cut into 1-inch segments, white and green parts
- 1 teaspoon sea salt
- 1 teaspoon white pepper

Heat a skillet over medium heat and when hot, cook the chicken and 1 tablespoon of the vegetable broth for about 5 minutes or until the chicken is lightly browned. Add the remaining 3 tablespoons vegetable broth and the mustard greens, mushrooms, garlic, ginger, and vinegar. Cover and cook for 5 minutes to give the greens time to soften just a little. Remove from the heat and stir in the green onions, salt, and pepper and serve.

* Marinated Chicken and Veggie Kabobs SERVES 1

PREP TIME: 10 minutes ▪ **TOTAL TIME:** about 4 hours

4 ounces boneless, skinless chicken breast

1 onion

½ teaspoon sea salt

½ teaspoon pepper

¼ cup any Phase 2 dressing

½ cup cubed (1½-inch pieces) red bell peppers

6 small whole button or cremini mushrooms

1 cup steamed spinach

1. Cut the chicken into 1½-inch pieces. Cut the onion into 6 small wedges. Put both the chicken and the onions in a bowl. Stir the salt and pepper into the dressing and pour over the chicken and onions. Toss gently to coat and then cover the bowl and refrigerate for at least 4 hours and up to 8 hours to marinate.

2. Thread the meat, onions, peppers, and mushrooms on metal skewers and grill over medium heat for 10 minutes, or until chicken is cooked through and vegetables are tender.

3. Serve on a bed of steamed spinach.

Long and Slow Beef Stew SERVES 8

PREP TIME: 10 minutes ▪ **TOTAL TIME:** 3 to 8 hours (slow cooker)

2 pounds diced beef stewing meat

¼ cup arrowroot

2 cups shredded cabbage

1 cup diced celery

1 cup green beans, cut in small pieces

1 cup quartered mushrooms

½ cup diced green onions (scallions), white and green parts

½ cup diced onion

1 tablespoon sea salt

½ teaspoon dried thyme

1 bay leaf

4 cups organic beef broth

1. Set a large pan on high heat. Sear the beef until its edges are nicely browned.

2. Slide the meat into a slow cooker, making sure to scrape up the brown bits in the pan. Add the rest of the ingredients to the slow cooker, and cook for 3 to 4 hours on high or 6 to 8 hours on low. Remove bay leaf when done and serve piping hot.

Turkey Meat Loaf and Asparagus SERVES 8

PREP TIME: 10 minutes ■ **TOTAL TIME:** 1 hour 20 minutes

2 pounds ground turkey

½ cup diced onion

½ cup chopped celery

2 large egg whites or ⅓ cup liquid egg whites

2 tablespoons coconut aminos

1 teaspoon minced garlic

1 teaspoon sea salt

1 teaspoon black pepper

2 pounds steamed asparagus

1. Preheat the oven to 375°F.

2. Combine all ingredients except the asparagus in a large mixing bowl. Press the mixture into a nonstick loaf pan and bake for about 1 hour. Let rest for 10 minutes. Slice and serve with asparagus.

Baked Cod and Veggies SERVES 4

PREP TIME: 5 minutes ■ **TOTAL TIME:** 30 minutes

2 cups asparagus spears, tough stems discarded, cut into 1-inch lengths

1 cup chopped broccoli

2 tablespoons tamari

1½ pounds fresh cod

1 lemon, sliced

1 tablespoon paprika

¼ teaspoon sea salt

⅛ teaspoon dry mustard

Pinch of fresh dill weed

1. Preheat the oven to 450°F.

2. Put the asparagus and broccoli in an oven-safe baking dish, sprinkle with tamari, cover with aluminum foil, and bake for 10 to 15 minutes or until the vegetables soften. Put the cod on top of the vegetables and top the fish with the lemon slices. Season with paprika, salt, mustard, and dill. Cover with the foil and bake for 10 to 15 minutes longer or until the cod is cooked through.

Steak Fajita Lettuce Wraps SERVES 4

PREP TIME: 10 minutes ▪ **TOTAL TIME:** 18 minutes

1 pound skirt steak, sliced into ½-inch strips

2 tablespoons organic vegetable broth

1 red bell pepper, seeded and thinly sliced

1 yellow bell pepper, seeded and thinly sliced

1 Vidalia onion, thinly sliced

1 cup sliced mushrooms

4 garlic cloves, minced

1 teaspoon chopped chipotle pepper

1 tablespoon chopped fresh cilantro

1 teaspoon crushed red pepper flakes

3 tablespoons fresh lime juice

1 head of lettuce, large leaves separated to use as cups

Heat a heavy-bottomed skillet over medium heat and when hot, sear the skirt steak, stirring often, for about 3 minutes, or until lightly browned. Add the broth, bell peppers, onion, mushrooms, garlic, chipotle pepper, cilantro, and red pepper flakes and stir well. Sprinkle with lime juice, stir again and cook for about 5 minutes longer, stirring, until the steak is cooked through or cooked to the desired degree of doneness. Spoon the steak filling into lettuce cups and serve immediately.

TIP: My favorite lettuce to use for these yummy wraps is Bibb lettuce.

Rosemary Pork Tenderloin with Mustard Greens SERVES 8

PREP TIME: 5 minutes ■ **TOTAL TIME:** 40 minutes to 24 hours (depending on length of marinating time)

2 pounds pork tenderloin

2 tablespoons finely chopped fresh rosemary leaves

6 tablespoons whole-grain, seedy mustard

6 tablespoons coconut vinegar

1 teaspoon vanilla extract

¼ teaspoon ground cinnamon

4 cups mustard greens

1. Put the pork in a shallow glass, ceramic, or other nonreactive dish. In a small bowl, stir together the rosemary, mustard, vinegar, vanilla extract, and cinnamon. Pour the marinade over the pork, cover, and refrigerate for at least 15 minutes and up to 24 hours.

2. Preheat the broiler.

3. Transfer the pork to a broiling pan and broil 4 to 6 inches from the heat for 7 to 8 minutes. Turn the pork over, baste, and broil for about 7 minutes longer or until the meat is cooked through. Transfer the pork to a cutting board and let it rest for 10 minutes before slicing.

4. Steam mustard greens for 3 to 5 minutes. Cut the pork into ¾-inch-thick slices and put on top of the steamed greens. Drizzle a tablespoon of the pan juices over each serving.

Sardine Salad with Kale and Bacon SERVES 2

PREP TIME: 5 minutes **TOTAL TIME:** 35 minutes

4 slices turkey bacon, chopped

3 garlic cloves, minced

Bunch of kale, ribs removed and leaves roughly chopped

Black pepper to taste

½ cup organic chicken broth

2 3-ounce cans smoked sardines in water, drained

In a skillet over low heat, sauté the bacon for about 4 minutes on each side, until it begins to brown. Raise th e heat to medium and add the garlic. Sauté for about 1 minute, then add the kale and pepper and toss and cook for about 4 minutes, until the kale begins to wilt. Add the broth and ½ cup of water, raise the heat slightly, and simmer for about 15 minutes or until the kale is just cooked and most of the liquid is evaporated. Add the sardines, mix well, and serve warm.

Lemon Mustard Pepper Chicken SERVES 8

PREP TIME: 10 minutes ∎ **TOTAL TIME:** 3 to 8 hours (slow cooker)

- 2 pounds boneless, skinless chicken breast, diced into 2-inch pieces
- 1 red bell pepper, seeded and diced
- 1 yellow bell pepper, seeded and diced
- 1 orange bell pepper, seeded and diced

- 2 cups organic chicken broth
- ¾ cup Dijon mustard
- ¼ cup diced red onion
- ¼ cup birch xylitol
- 2 tablespoons coconut aminos
- 2 sprigs fresh rosemary
- Juice of 1 lemon

Put all ingredients into a slow cooker or Crock-Pot and cook for 3 to 4 hours on high or 6 to 8 hours on low. Remove the rosemary sprigs before serving.

TIP: All of the dinners on Phase 2 can also be eaten as a lunch. One of my favorite things to do is take the leftovers from this dinner and serve over a bed of mixed greens with Phase 2 dressing and then eat it for tomorrow's Phase 2 lunch.

Greek Meatballs and Veggies SERVES 4

PREP TIME: 15 minutes ■ **TOTAL TIME:** 30 minutes

MEATBALLS:

- 1 pound ground lamb
- 2 garlic cloves, minced
- 1 large shallot, minced
- 1 tablespoon seeded, diced jalapeño pepper
- 2 tablespoons chopped fresh mint
- 1 tablespoon coconut aminos
- ½ teaspoon black pepper

VEGGIES:

- 1 red bell pepper, seeded and diced
- 1 green bell pepper, seeded and diced
- 1 onion, sliced
- 20 medium-sized mushrooms, sliced
- ½ cup arugula
- ¼ cup organic vegetable broth
- 1 tablespoon coconut aminos
- 1 teaspoon sea salt
- ½ teaspoon fresh or dried basil
- ¼ teaspoon fresh or dried dill weed
- ¼ teaspoon dried fennel
- ¼ teaspoon dried marjoram

1. For the meatballs: Preheat the oven to 375°F.

2. Mix all the ingredients for the meatballs in a bowl. Between dampened palms, roll the meat into meatballs that are about 2 inches in diameter. As they are made, put the meatballs in an oven-proof dish. Cover with aluminum foil and bake for about 20 minutes or until the meatballs are cooked through. While the meatballs are baking, make the veggies.

3. For the veggies: In a large sauté pan, sauté the vegetables, broth, aminos, salt, and herbs over medium-high heat for about 15 minutes or until the peppers are tender. Serve the veggies with the meatballs.

TIP: My favorite mushroom to use in this recipe is shiitake because of the strong flavor, but any mushroom would be delicious.

New York Strip Steak with Broccoli SERVES 2

PREP TIME: 2 minutes ■ **TOTAL TIME:** 10 minutes

STEAK:

1 tablespoon minced garlic

½ teaspoon chopped fresh cilantro

¼ teaspoon sea salt

⅛ teaspoon fresh lemon juice

8 ounces New York strip steak

BROCCOLI:

2 cups broccoli florets

1 tablespoon fresh lemon juice

½ teaspoon brewer's yeast

1. Preheat the broiler to high.

2. For the steak: In a small bowl, combine the garlic, cilantro, salt, and lemon juice. Spread over the steak and broil for 3 to 4 minutes on each side or until the steak reaches the desired degree of doneness. Transfer the steak to a cutting board and let the meat rest for about 5 minutes before slicing.

3. For the broccoli: Fill the bottom of a steamer with water. Place the broccoli in the top part of the steamer, bring to a boil over high heat, reduce to a simmer, cover tightly, and steam for about 5 minutes or until the desired doneness. Combine the lemon juice and brewer's yeast and dress the broccoli. Serve with the steak.

Edamame and Leek Salad SERVES 1

PREP TIME: 5 minutes ▪ **TOTAL TIME:** 10 minutes

2 large leeks, cleaned and trimmed

½ cup cooked edamame

¼ cup organic vegetable broth

3 tablespoons coconut vinegar

1 teaspoon birch xylitol

1 teaspoon mustard seeds

1 teaspoon lemon juice

Cut the leeks into ½-inch-thick slices. Bring a pot of water to a simmer over medium-high heat and cook the leeks for about 5 minutes or until just tender. Drain and transfer to a shallow serving bowl. Add the edamame and toss. In a small bowl, whisk together the broth, vinegar, xylitol, mustard seeds, and lemon juice. Pour over the leeks and toss to mix.

TIP: I love to convert leftovers from this dinner by puréeing it in a blender and serving it as a hot soup. The soup also freezes really well and can be saved for a Phase 2 lunch or dinner.

NOTE: Because it contains edamame (soy beans), this recipe is only for vegans or vegetarians who do not eat eggs.

Tempeh Vegetable Stew SERVES 2

PREP TIME: 10 minutes ■ TOTAL TIME: 3 to 8 hours (slow cooker)

8 ounces tempeh, cut into 1-inch cubes

2 cups broccoli florets

2 cups shredded cabbage

1 cup kale, ribs removed and leaves roughly chopped

1 cup sliced leeks

¼ cup diced celery

¼ cup diced red onion

1 dried bay leaf

4 cups organic vegetable broth

2 tablespoons coconut aminos

1 tablespoon minced garlic

1 teaspoon sea salt

½ teaspoon dried basil

½ teaspoon turmeric

Put all the ingredients into a slow cooker or Crock-Pot and cook for 3 to 4 hours on high or 6 to 8 hours on low. Remove the bay leaf before serving.

NOTE: Because it contains tempeh, this recipe is only for vegans or vegetarians who do not eat eggs.

Portobello Mushrooms and Mustard Greens SERVES 4

PREP TIME: 5 minutes ■ TOTAL TIME: 10 minutes

Bunch of mustard greens, roughly chopped

2 cups portobello mushrooms, stemmed and chopped

4 garlic cloves

1 tablespoon coconut vinegar

¼ cup organic vegetable broth

1 15-ounce can white beans

Bunch of green onions (scallions), cut into 1-inch slices, white and green parts

1 tablespoon minced ginger

1 teaspoon sea salt

1 teaspoon white pepper

Heat a large skillet over medium heat and when hot, cook the mustard greens, mushrooms, garlic, and vinegar with the broth for about 1 minute, stirring. Cover the skillet and continue to cook for 5 to 6 minutes longer or until the vegetables are soft. Remove from the heat; add the white beans, green onions, ginger, salt, and white pepper, and serve.

TIP: I use portobello mushrooms in this recipe because they not only contain protein, but have more potassium than a banana. Combined with the mustard greens, this meal is a natural diuretic.

Garden Egg White * Scramble SERVES 1

PREP TIME: 5 minutes ■ TOTAL TIME: 10 minutes

½ cup chopped mushrooms

1 tablespoon chopped onion

1 tablespoon chopped shallot

1 tablespoon minced garlic

1 tablespoon minced green chile

1 cup chopped leeks

3 large egg whites or ½ cup liquid egg whites

1 teaspoon chopped fresh parsley or cilantro

¼ teaspoon crushed red pepper flakes

Pinch of sea salt

1. In a nonstick pan, heat 1 teaspoon of water over medium-high heat and cook the mushrooms, onion, shallot, garlic, and green chile until soft. Stir in the leeks and cook until wilted. Add the egg whites and stir until scrambled. Allow the eggs to cook until desired consistency.

2. Sprinkle with parsley, red pepper flakes, and salt before serving.

Three-Pepper Egg White Soufflé SERVES 2

PREP TIME: 10 minutes ■ **TOTAL TIME:** 35 to 40 minutes

2 tablespoons organic vegetable broth

½ cup diced red bell pepper

½ cup diced yellow bell pepper

¼ cup diced yellow onion

½ teaspoon cayenne pepper

6 large egg whites, at room temperature, or 1 cup liquid egg whites

1 teaspoon fresh lemon juice

Sea salt and black pepper to taste

1. Preheat the oven to 350°F.

2. Heat a skillet over medium heat and when hot, add the broth and sauté the bell peppers and onion until soft. Stir in the cayenne pepper. Whisk the egg whites and lemon juice until stiff peaks form using a wire whisk or an electric mixer. Gently fold the pepper-and-onion mixture into the egg whites and pour the mixture into a 9-inch nonstick baking pan. Working quickly but steadily, smooth the surface and bake for 25 to 30 minutes, or until the top is golden brown and a knife inserted in the middle comes out clean. Season with salt and pepper to taste and serve immediately.

Mustard Egg Salad ✗ SERVES 2

PREP TIME: 5 minutes ▪ **TOTAL TIME:** 5 minutes

¼ cup diced celery

3 tablespoons spicy mustard

½ teaspoon fresh lemon juice

Pinch of fresh dill weed

3 large hard-cooked egg whites, chopped

In a small bowl, stir together the celery, mustard, lemon juice, and dill weed. Fold the egg whites into the celery mixture and serve.

Roast Beef–Wrapped Pickles SERVES 1

PREP TIME: 2 minutes ▪ **TOTAL TIME:** 2 minutes

2 ounces nitrate-free sliced roast beef, cut into 4 slices

4 dill pickle spears, no preservatives, no sugars added

Roll the roast beef around the pickle spears and enjoy. Feel free to add mustard or horseradish if you like.

TIP: We only use 2 ounces of roast beef in this recipe because remember that in Phase 2, we halve the normal protein portion (2 ounces instead of 4) for snacks.

Smoked Salmon and Celery SERVES 1

PREP TIME: 2 minutes ■ **TOTAL TIME:** 2 minutes

Fresh lemon juice to taste

4 celery stalks

Sea salt to taste

3 ounces smoked salmon, nitrate-free, no sugar added

Squeeze lemon juice on the celery stalks and sprinkle with sea salt. Serve with the salmon.

TIP: Make sure salmon is nitrate free.

Wild Sardine Pâté SERVES 1

PREP TIME: 2 minutes ■ **TOTAL TIME:** 2 minutes

1 3¾-ounce can wild sardines packed in water

1 teaspoon Dijon mustard

Celery sticks

Put the sardines (with the water) and mustard in a food processor and pulse several times until a smooth pâté forms. Stuff the celery sticks with the pâté or use it as a dip.

Red Pepper Stuffed with Crunchy Tuna Salad *

SERVES 1

PREP TIME: 2 minutes ▪ **TOTAL TIME:** 2 minutes

3 to 3½ ounces water-packed tuna, drained

¼ cup diced dill pickles

¼ cup diced celery

3 tablespoons spicy mustard

Pinch of fresh dill weed

½ teaspoon fresh lemon juice

½ red bell pepper (bottom half), seeded

In a small bowl, mix together the tuna, pickles, celery, mustard, dill weed, and lemon juice and mix well. Stuff the tuna mixture into the bell pepper and serve.

TIP: I like to save the second half of the bell pepper to slice up and eat for a snack, but if you are still hungry, have at it.

Garden Meatballs SERVES 12

(OR 6 DINNERS)

PREP TIME: 10 minutes ▪ TOTAL TIME: 45 minutes

½ pound lean ground turkey

1 pound lean ground beef

4 cups spinach, finely chopped

½ cup finely chopped celery

4 green onions (scallions), finely chopped, white and green parts

1 bell pepper, seeded and finely diced

⅓ cup chile paste thinned with 2 tablespoons Bragg's Liquid Aminos

2 7-ounce cans diced mild green chiles

1 teaspoon sea salt, or to taste

½ teaspoon black pepper

1. Preheat the oven to 375°F.

2. In a large mixing bowl, combine all the ingredients. With dampened palms, roll the meat mixture into meatballs and transfer them to a 9 × 13-inch baking dish (or larger, depending on the size of meatballs). Bake for 25 to 35 minutes, turning the meatballs over after 15 minutes, or until the meatballs are cooked through. Remove from the oven and cool. Serve warm or room temperature, or store to serve later.

3. These meatballs may be prepared in advance and frozen in freezer bags, divided evenly among 12 bags. On the day you plan to use them, thaw them in the refrigerator. They can be eaten cold or slightly warmed.

TIP: I like to make a big batch of these because they freeze really well and I can keep them on hand for snacks. I freeze them in snack portions (about 2 ounces) in ziplock bags, and then if I'm going to eat them for dinner I'll just defrost two of them.

Summer Salsa with Turkey Bacon Chips ✗ SERVES 2

PREP TIME: 10 minutes ▪ **TOTAL TIME:** overnight (to marinate) plus 40 minutes cook time

1 pound fresh asparagus spears, tough stems removed, cut into ½-inch lengths

1 cup chopped fresh cucumber

½ cup finely chopped onion

1 tablespoon chopped fresh cilantro

1 jalapeño pepper, seeded and finely chopped

1½ teaspoons apple cider vinegar

½ teaspoon sea salt

4 ounces turkey bacon

1. Put the asparagus in a large saucepan with 2 cups water, bring to a boil over medium-high heat, cover, reduce heat, and cook for about 2 minutes. Drain and rinse in cold water. Transfer to a mixing bowl and add the cucumber, onion, cilantro, jalapeño, vinegar, and salt. Cover and refrigerate for 4 to 5 hours or overnight.

2. Preheat the oven to 375°F.

3. Lay the bacon strips in a baking dish large enough to hold them in a single layer and bake for about 20 minutes. Poke the bacon with the tines of a fork several times during baking to keep it flat. Drain the bacon on paper towels and when cool, cut into chip-size pieces with kitchen scissors. Serve the bacon with the salsa.

Leftover Lettuce Cups with Dressing SERVES 1

PREP TIME: 2 minutes ▪ **TOTAL TIME:** 2 minutes

1 cup of protein leftovers from any Phase 2 dinner

1 lettuce cup

Any Phase 2 dressing

Stuff the leftovers into the lettuce cup and drizzle with any Phase 2 dressing.

Oysters on Cucumbers SERVES 1

PREP TIME: 2 minutes ▪ **TOTAL TIME:** 2 minutes

1 3¾-ounce can smoked oysters, packed in water

½ cup sliced cucumbers

Fresh lime juice or any Phase 2 dressing (optional)

Set the oysters on the cucumber slices. Dress with lime juice or any Phase 2 dressing, if using. Serve immediately.

Salty Edamame SERVES 2

PREP TIME: 2 minutes ■ **TOTAL TIME:** 5 minutes

1 cup edamame, in their pods	**Sea salt and crushed red pepper flakes to taste**

Steam the edamame in their pods for about 3 minutes. While still warm, sprinkle with salt and red pepper flakes. Eat right away or when cool.

NOTE: Because it contains edamame (soy beans), this recipe is only for vegans or vegetarians who do not eat eggs.

Sardine and Cucumber Canapés SERVES 1

PREP TIME: 2 minutes ■ **TOTAL TIME:** 2 minutes

1 3-ounce can sardines, packed in water, drained	**1 teaspoon lemon juice**
⅛ teaspoon cayenne pepper	**1 cucumber, sliced**

In a small bowl, combine the sardines, cayenne pepper, and lemon juice and mix with a fork, breaking up the fish as it mixes with the pepper and lemon juice. Top the cucumber slices with the sardine mixture.

Peppery Tofu Jerky **SERVES 8**

PREP TIME: 5 minutes ■ **TOTAL TIME:** 20 hours

16 ounces firm or extra-firm tofu

½ cup tamari

3 tablespoons liquid smoke

1 tablespoon onion powder

1 teaspoon minced garlic

10 drops liquid stevia

1 tablespoon black pepper

1. Cut the tofu widthwise into 12 thin slices. Put the tamari, liquid smoke, onion powder, minced garlic, stevia, and pepper in a gallon-size plastic food storage bag and add 2 tablespoons of water. Shake the bag a little to mix the ingredients together. Add the tofu slices, shake the bag to coat the tofu, seal tightly, and refrigerate for at least 12 hours.

2. Preheat the oven to 170°F.

3. Lift the tofu from the marinade, letting any excess drip back into the bag. Lay the slices on a parchment-lined baking sheet and bake for about 7 hours, or until they are very dry, or reach the desired texture. You can also use a dehydrator. Serve cold.

NOTE: Because it contains tofu, this recipe is only for vegans or vegetarians who do not eat eggs.

Arnold Palmer SERVES 1

PREP TIME: 2 minutes ■ **TOTAL TIME:** 5 minutes

1 peppermint tea bag

1 chamomile tea bag

Juice of ½ lemon
(2 tablespoons)

¼ cup birch xylitol

Brew the tea bags in a large mug of hot water. Pour the tea over a glass of ice and add the lemon juice and xylitol. Stir to mix and serve right away.

Lime-Mint Smoothie SERVES 1

PREP TIME: 2 minutes ■ **TOTAL TIME:** 2 minutes

2 cups ice cubes

½ cup peeled, diced lime

1 fresh mint leaf

Birch xylitol to taste

Blend the ingredients plus ½ cup of water until smooth. Serve right away.

Homemade Lemonade SERVES 3 TO 6

PREP TIME: 2 minutes ▪ **TOTAL TIME:** 2 minutes

1 cup fresh lemon juice

¾ cup birch xylitol

Sliced lemon for garnish, optional

Combine the lemon juice and xylitol with 5 cups of water in a pitcher and stir well. Serve over ice and garnish with sliced lemon, if desired.

Colon Cleanse Smoothie SERVES 1

PREP TIME: 5 minutes ▪ **TOTAL TIME:** 5 minutes

½ cup chopped spinach

½ cup chopped celery

¼ head cabbage

1 lime, peeled

1 cup ice cubes

½ cup brewed senna tea

Blend the ingredients plus 1 cup of water until smooth. Serve right away.

TIP: It's a good idea to chop your cabbage before blending it if you're not using a high-speed blender.

TIP: Sometimes protein can cause constipation; it is very important to make sure the bowels move.

Detox Smoothie SERVES 1

PREP TIME: 2 minutes ■ **TOTAL TIME:** 2 minutes

½ cup kale, ribs removed and coarsely chopped

½ cup peeled, diced cucumber

½ teaspoon chopped fresh parsley

½ teaspoon minced ginger

1 cup ice cubes

1 heaping tablespoon spirulina

Blend the ingredients plus 2 cups of water until smooth. Serve right away.

TIP: This is great for acne and detoxing the liver.

TIP: Spirulina is a protein-rich food that can be found at your local health food store or online.

Sun Tea Mojito SERVES 1

PREP TIME: 2 minutes ■ **TOTAL TIME:** 2 minutes

1 tablespoon fresh lime juice

1 fresh mint leaf

1 teaspoon birch xylitol

1 cup sun tea, such as Smooth Move, senna, or chamomile

Stir together all ingredients and serve over ice.

One serving for all dips and dressings is 2 to 4 tablespoons.

Red Bell Pepper Dressing SERVES 4 TO 6

PREP TIME: 5 minutes ▪ **TOTAL TIME:** 5 minutes

½ red bell pepper, seeded and chopped

1 teaspoon chopped fresh cilantro

1 tablespoon tamari

1 teaspoon sea salt

½ teaspoon arrowroot powder

½ teaspoon dry mustard

½ teaspoon black pepper

Blend the ingredients with ½ cup of water until smooth. Serve over any Phase 2 salad or as a dip with any raw Phase 2 veggies.

TIP: Feel free to use prepared mustard in this recipe, as long as it doesn't include sugar or artificial ingredients.

Pepperoncini Dressing SERVES 2 TO 4

PREP TIME: 2 minutes ■ **TOTAL TIME:** 2 minutes

¼ cup pepperoncini in juice

¼ cup fresh lime juice

1 tablespoon crushed red pepper flakes

1 tablespoon chopped fresh cilantro

5 drops stevia

Blend the ingredients with ½ cup of water until smooth. Serve over any Phase 2 salad or drizzle over any Phase 2 veggies.

TIP: I'm a huge fan of flavored stevias. I love to use Valencia orange stevia for this recipe. You can find it at your local health food store or online.

Lemon Vinaigrette SERVES 2 TO 4

PREP TIME: 2 minutes ■ **TOTAL TIME:** 2 minutes

¼ cup coconut vinegar

1 teaspoon stevia

1 tablespoon fresh lemon juice

Put all ingredients in a food processor or blender and blend until smooth, or whisk together in a small bowl. Serve over any Phase 2 salad or drizzle over any Phase 2 veggies.

TIP: I often find myself making these dressings by simply whisking them in a bowl with a fork. No blender needed!

Chipotle Dressing SERVES APPROXIMATELY 2

PREP TIME: 5 minutes ■ **TOTAL TIME:** 5 minutes

2 tablespoons fresh lime juice

2 tablespoons coconut vinegar

2 teaspoons grated lime zest

1 teaspoon dry mustard

1 teaspoon ground chipotle powder

¼ teaspoon ground cumin

¼ teaspoon chili powder

¼ teaspoon fresh or dried oregano

⅛ teaspoon stevia

⅛ teaspoon paprika

Blend the ingredients until smooth. Serve right away. Serve over any Phase 2 salad, meal, or veggies.

Fiery Southwestern Dip SERVES APPROXIMATELY 2

PREP TIME: 2 minutes ■ **TOTAL TIME:** 2 minutes

⅓ cup coconut vinegar

2 tablespoons fresh lemon juice

4½ teaspoons birch xylitol

1 tablespoon ground cumin

1 tablespoon minced garlic

1 tablespoon tamari

1½ teaspoons crushed red pepper flakes

1½ teaspoons black pepper

1 teaspoon sea salt

½ teaspoon Tabasco sauce

Blend the ingredients until smooth. Serve over any Phase 2 salad or meal or as a dip with any raw Phase 2 veggies.

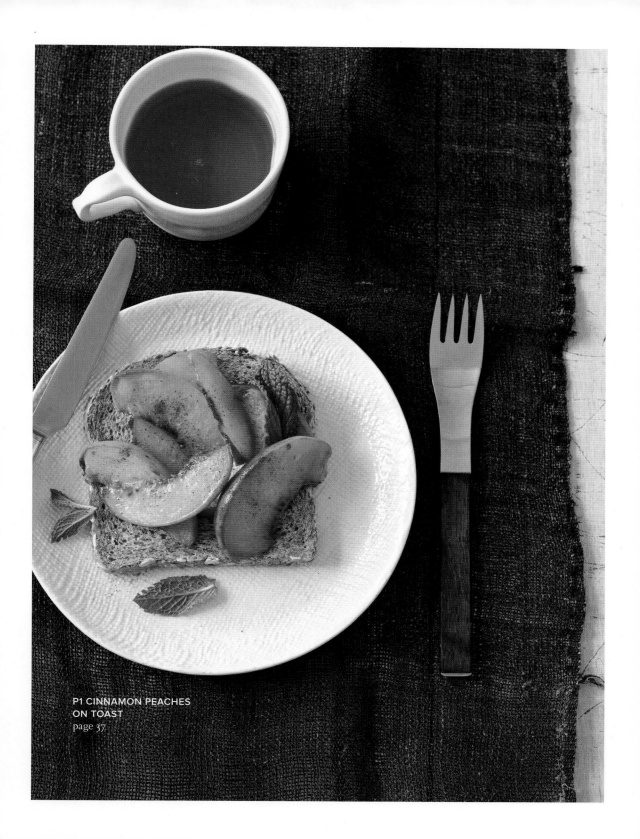

P1 CINNAMON PEACHES
ON TOAST
page 37

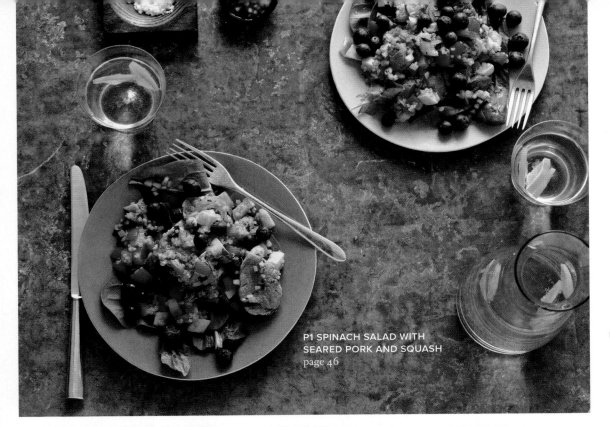

P1 SPINACH SALAD WITH
SEARED PORK AND SQUASH
page 46

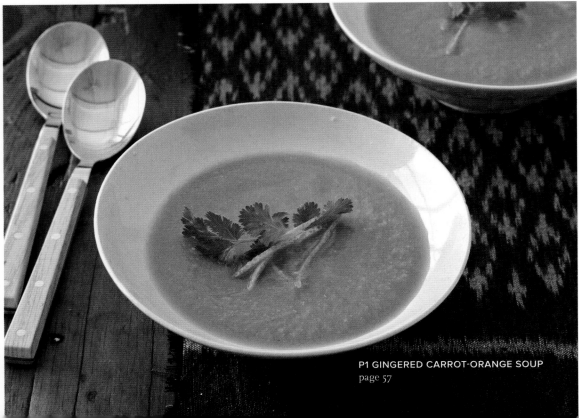

P1 GINGERED CARROT-ORANGE SOUP
page 57

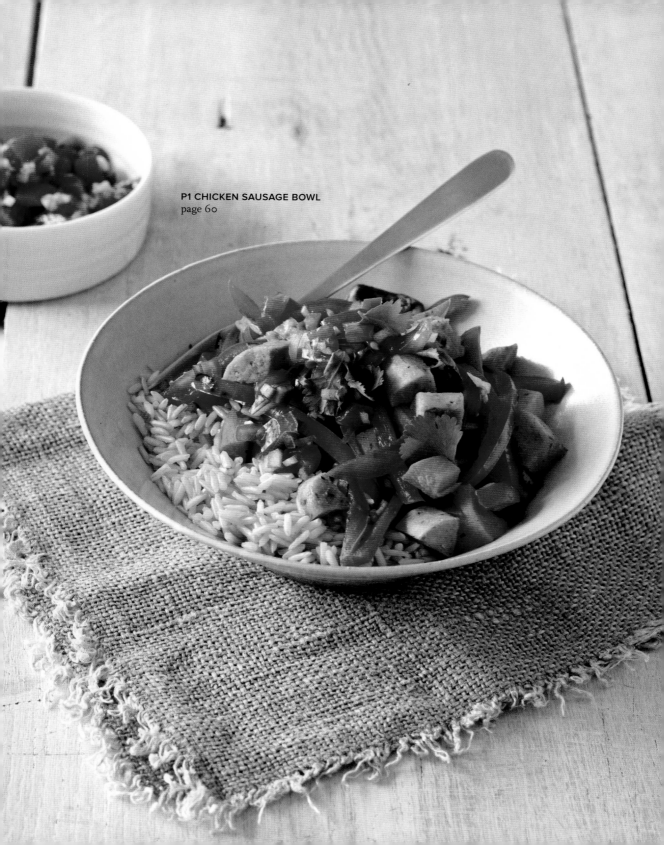

P1 CHICKEN SAUSAGE BOWL
page 60

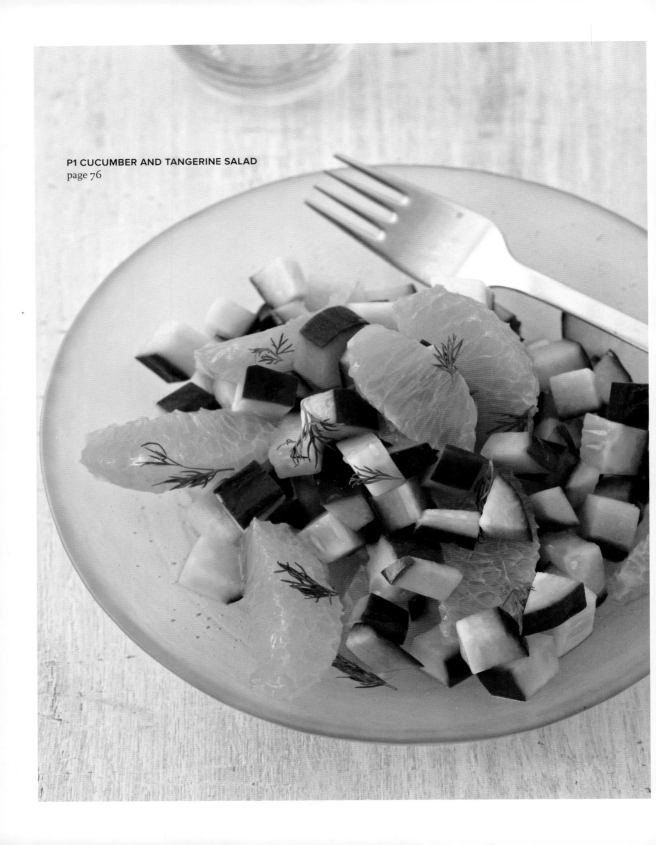

P1 CUCUMBER AND TANGERINE SALAD
page 76

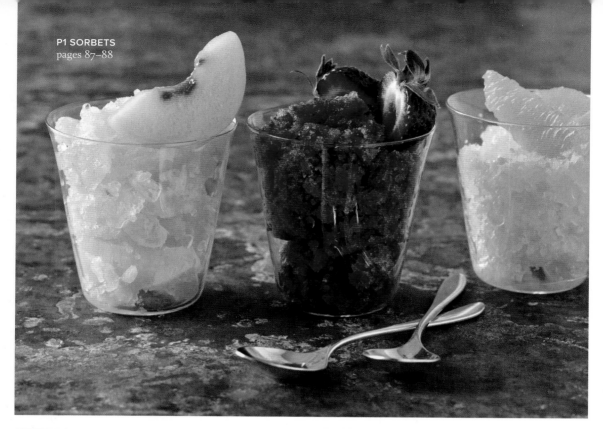

P1 SORBETS
pages 87–88

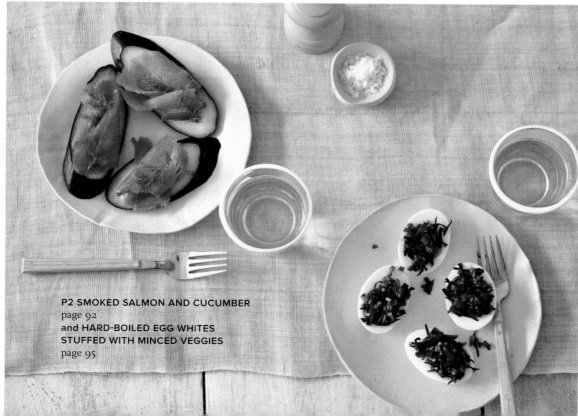

P2 SMOKED SALMON AND CUCUMBER
page 92
and **HARD-BOILED EGG WHITES
STUFFED WITH MINCED VEGGIES**
page 95

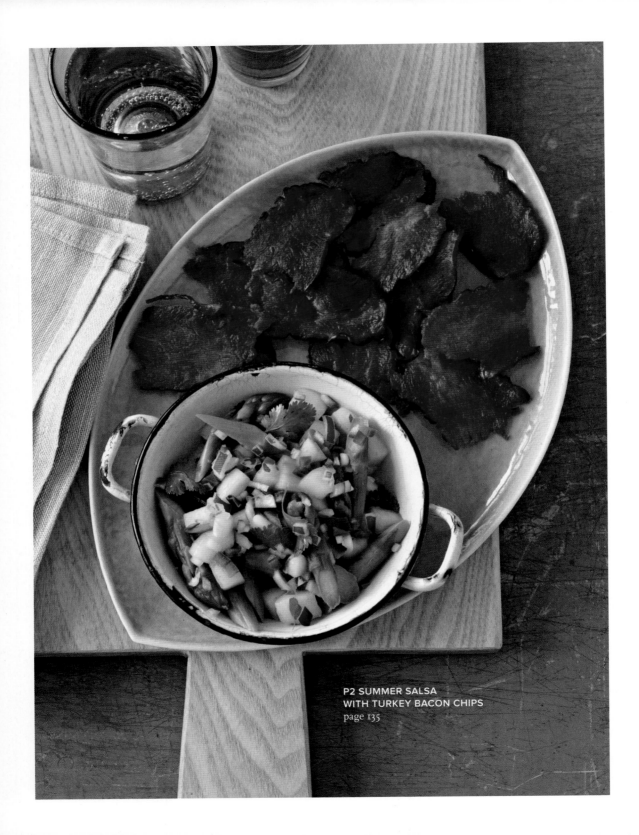

P2 SUMMER SALSA
WITH TURKEY BACON CHIPS
page 135

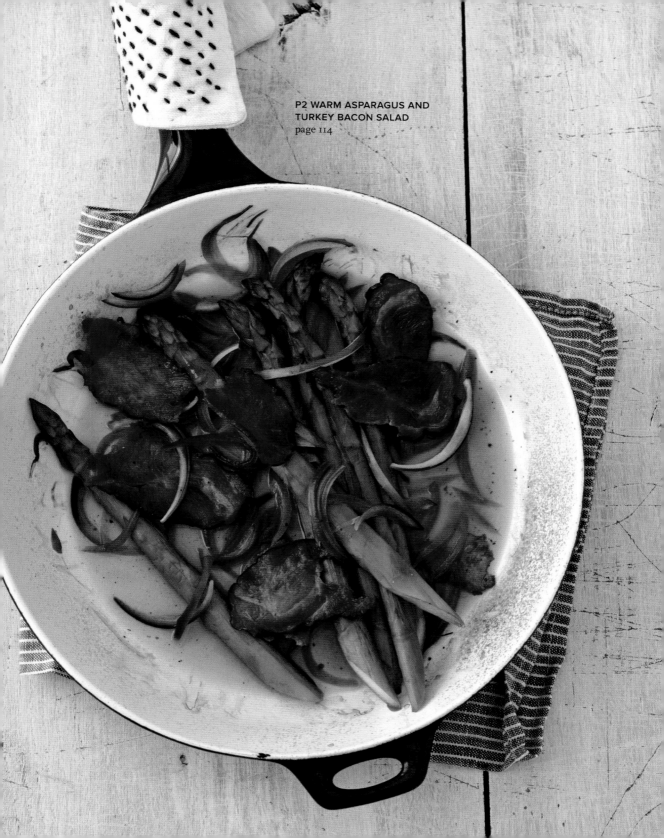

**P2 WARM ASPARAGUS AND
TURKEY BACON SALAD**
page 114

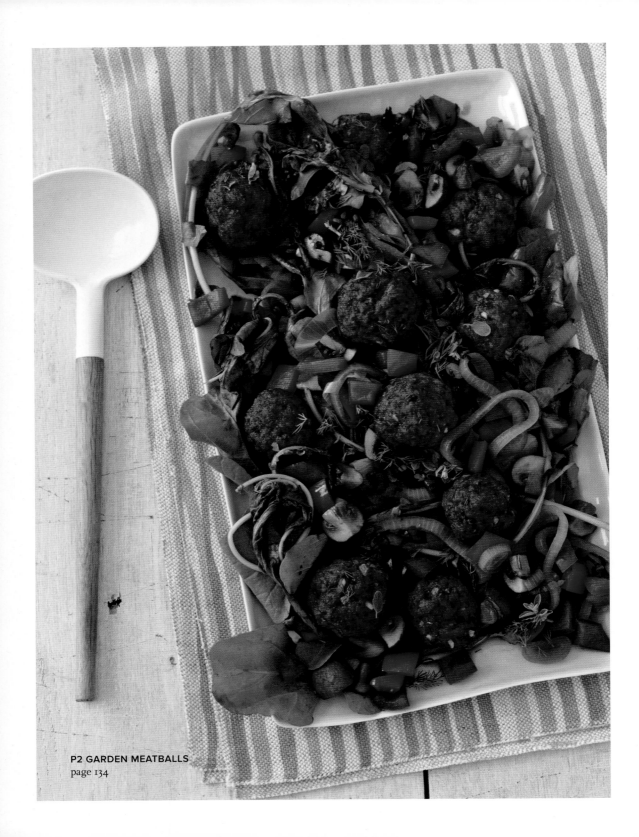

P2 GARDEN MEATBALLS
page 134

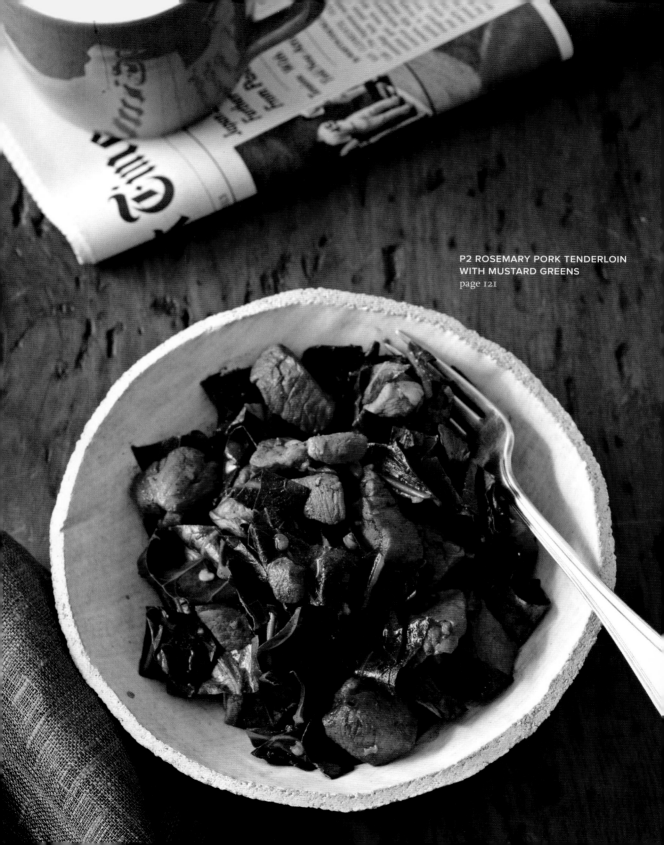

**P2 ROSEMARY PORK TENDERLOIN
WITH MUSTARD GREENS**
page 121

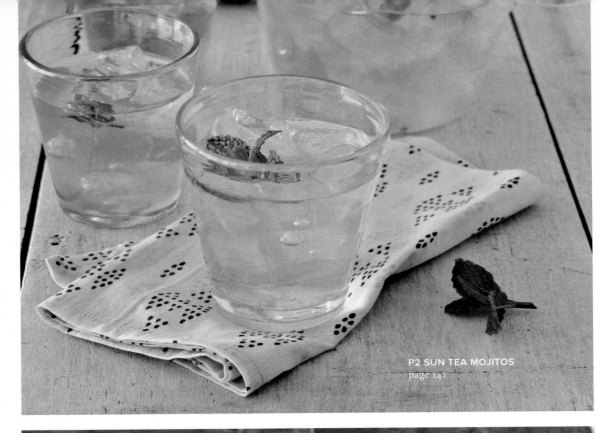

P2 SUN TEA MOJITOS
page 141

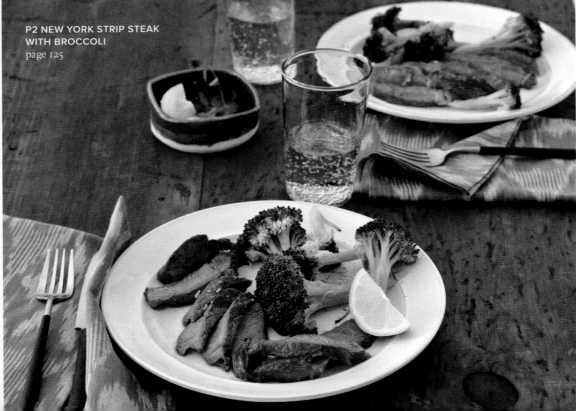

P2 NEW YORK STRIP STEAK WITH BROCCOLI
page 125

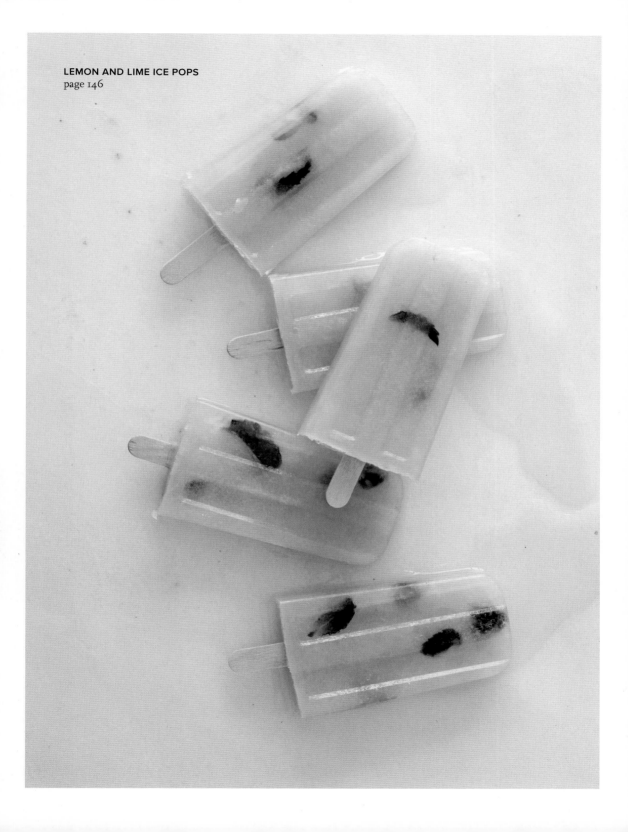

LEMON AND LIME ICE POPS
page 146

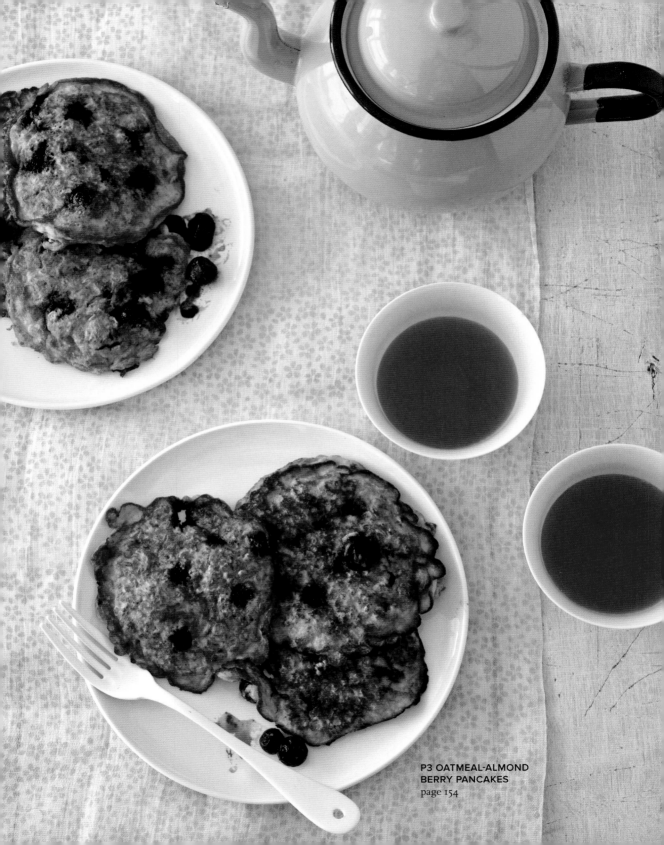

**P3 OATMEAL-ALMOND
BERRY PANCAKES**
page 154

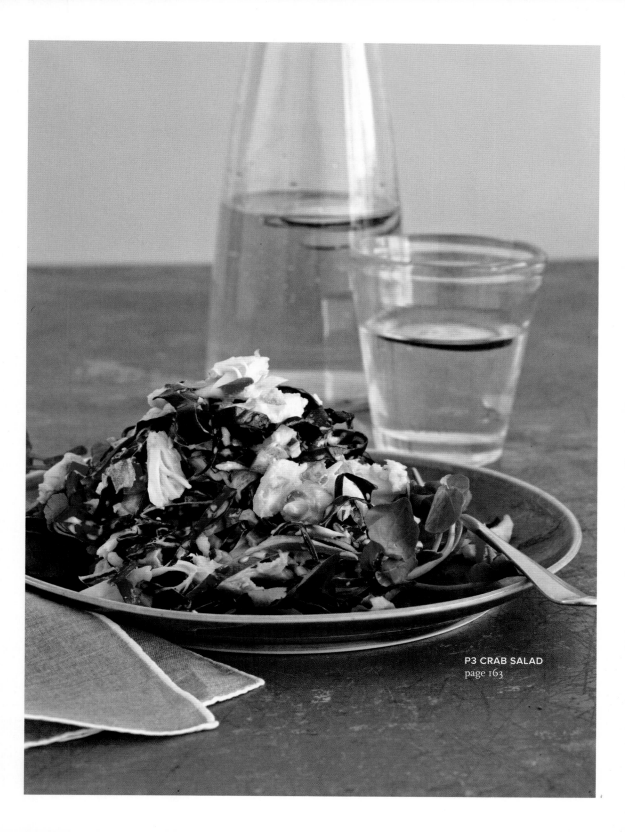

P3 CRAB SALAD
page 163

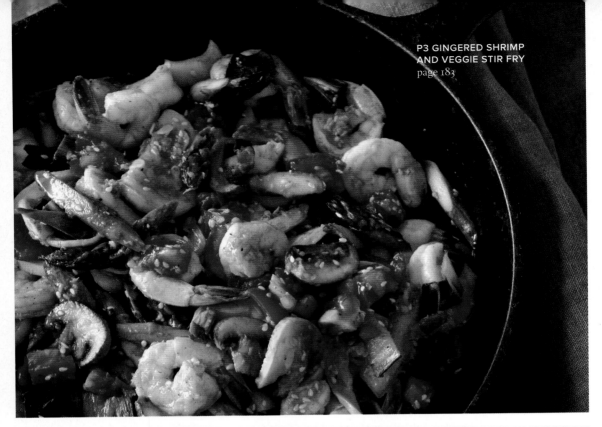

P3 GINGERED SHRIMP
AND VEGGIE STIR FRY
page 183

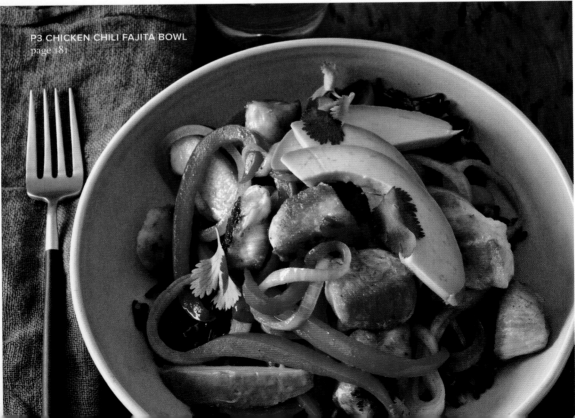

P3 CHICKEN CHILI FAJITA BOWL
page 181

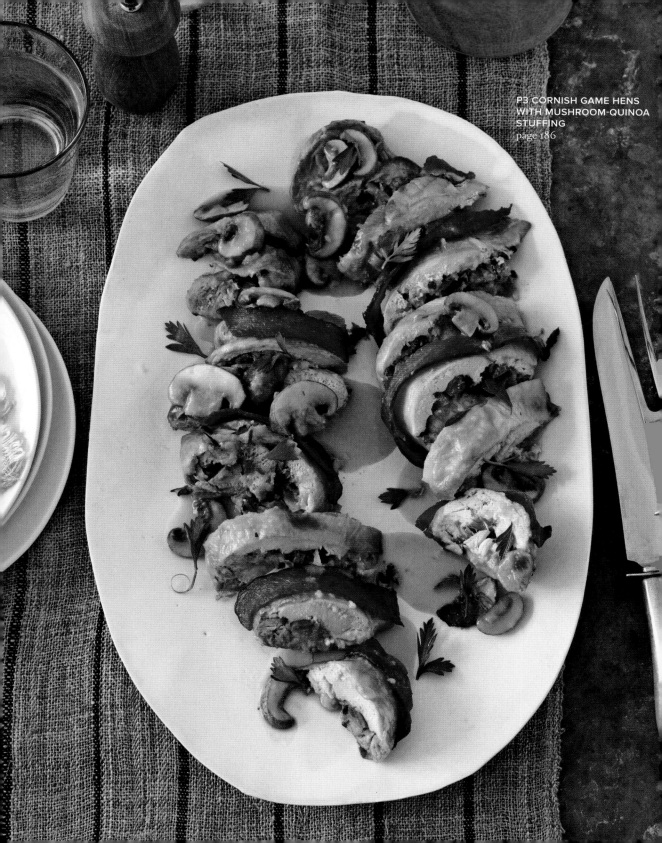

P3 CORNISH GAME HENS
WITH MUSHROOM-QUINOA
STUFFING
page 186

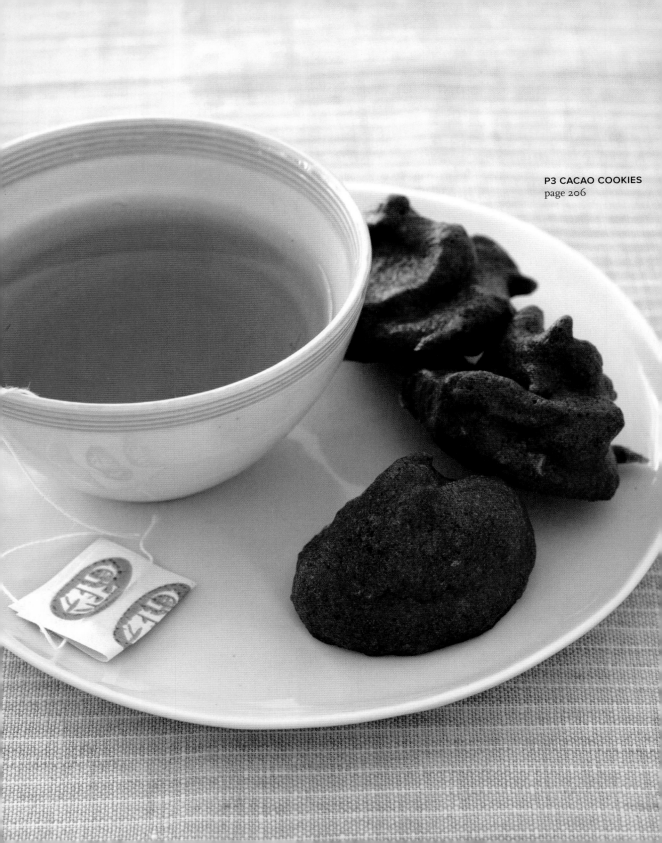

P3 CACAO COOKIES
page 206

Lime Sorbet SERVES 2

PREP TIME: 2 minutes ▪ TOTAL TIME: 2 minutes

1 cup chopped lettuce
1 lime, peeled

½ cup birch xylitol
4 cups ice cubes

Blend the ingredients until smooth. Add water as needed to thin. Serve right away.

TIP: Because lime and lemon are such low glycemic fruits, these treats can be eaten on any phase of the diet, with any meal, without adding a day of exercise.

Lemon Meringue SERVES 4 (1 SERVING IS 2 MERINGUES)

PREP TIME: 5 minutes ▪ TOTAL TIME: 4 hours

4 large egg whites or ⅔ cup liquid egg whites
½ teaspoon arrowroot powder

⅓ cup birch xylitol
2 tablespoons grated lemon zest

Line a baking sheet with parchment paper. In a glass bowl, whisk the egg whites and arrowroot until soft peaks form. Gradually add the xylitol and lemon zest, whisking until stiff peaks form. Spoon 8 meringues onto the baking sheet, mounding them into shape. Place in the oven at 200 degrees, propping the oven door open for several hours or until the meringues dry and harden. Enjoy immediately.

TIP: These yummy meringues contain protein, so you can eat them as a Phase 2 snack or with any Phase 2 meal if you add a day of exercise.

Lemon and Lime Ice Pops SERVES 1

PREP TIME: 2 minutes ▪ **TOTAL TIME:** 2 hours

¼ cup fresh lime juice

¼ cup birch xylitol

Juice of ½ lemon
(2 tablespoons)

1 fresh mint leaf

In a small bowl, whisk all ingredients together. Transfer to ice-pop molds or small paper cups. Freeze until frozen. Before the juice freezes solid and while it is still mushy, insert ice-pop sticks into the center of the ice pop. When ready to eat, release from the molds or tear off the paper and enjoy.

TIP: You can freeze these in ice-pop molds or simply in paper cups with a stick. When you are ready to eat, just tear the cup away and enjoy.

TIP: Because lime and lemon are such low glycemic fruits, these treats can be eaten on any phase of the diet, with any meal, without adding a day of exercise.

Phase 2 Food List

To modify any of the recipes for this phase of the diet, or to make up your own, you may use any of the foods on the following Phase 2 food list.

VEGETABLES AND SALAD GREENS (fresh, canned, or frozen)

Arrowroot

Arugula

Asparagus

Beans: *green, yellow (wax), French (string)*

Broccoli florets

Cabbage, all types

Celery

Collard greens

Cucumbers, any type

Endive

Fennel

Green chiles, jalapeños

Green onions

Jicama

Kale

Leeks

Lettuce (any except iceberg)

Mixed greens

Mushrooms

Mustard greens

Onions: *red, white, Vidalia, and yellow*

Peppers: *bell, pepperoncini*

Radishes

Rhubarb

Shallots

Spinach

Spirulina

Swiss chard

Watercress

FRUITS (fresh or frozen)

Lemons

Limes

ANIMAL PROTEIN

Beef, all lean cuts: *filet, tenderloin, strip, sirloin, shell steak, London broil, round steak, rump roast, skirt steak, stew meat, lean ground*

Buffalo meat

Chicken: *boneless, skinless white meat*

Cod/scrod fillet

Corned beef

Deli meats, nitrate-free: *roast beef, chicken, turkey*

Dory fish fillet

Eggs, whites only

Game: *venison, ostrich, elk*

Haddock fillet

Jerky, nitrate-free: *beef, buffalo, turkey, elk, ostrich*

Lamb, lean cuts, ground

Oysters, packed in water

Pork: *loin roast, tenderloin*

Salmon: *nitrate-free smoked*

Sardines, packed in water

Sole fillet

Tuna, fresh or packed in water

Turkey: *breast steaks, lean ground*

Turkey bacon: *nitrate-free*

VEGETABLE PROTEIN

None this phase

BROTHS, HERBS, SPICES, CONDIMENTS, AND SUPPLEMENTS

Brewer's yeast

Broths: *beef, chicken, vegetable**

Dried herbs: *all types*

Fresh herbs: *all types*

Garlic, fresh, powdered

Ginger, fresh

Horseradish, prepared

Mustard, prepared, dry

Natural seasonings: *Bragg Liquid Aminos, coconut amino acids, tamari*

Noncaffeinated herbal teas or Pero

Nutritional yeast

Pickles, no sugar added

Seasonings: *black and white peppers, cayenne, chili powder, chili paste, chipotle, cinnamon, crushed red pepper flakes, cumin, curry powder, lemon pepper, liquid smoke, nutmeg, onion powder, onion salt, paprika, raw cacao powder, sea salt*

Sweeteners: *stevia, xylitol (birch only)*

Tabasco

Vanilla or peppermint extract

Vinegar, any type (except rice)

GRAINS AND STARCHES

None this phase

HEALTHY FATS

None this phase

*NOTE: All broths, if possible, should be free of additives and preservatives.

PHASE 3

Breakfast

Cashew-Quinoa Hot Cereal
Avocado and Tomato on Toast
Black Bean and Tomato Toast
Spinach-Mushroom Omelet
Tomato-Topped Tuna Melt
Oatmeal-Almond Berry Pancakes
Breakfast Burrito
Peach-Coconut Tapioca
Raspberry-Studded Oatmeal
Fried Egg with Spinach
Almond Berry Pancakes
Sprouted-Grain Bagel with Smoked
Salmon
Dairy-Free Eggs Benedict

Lunch

Artichoke Salad with Avocado and
Hearts of Palm
Crab Salad
Avocado-Turkey Lettuce Wrap
Salmon Salad
Slow-Cooked Chicken Curry
Coconut Chicken with Butternut
Squash
Shrimp and Avocado Salad
Steak Fajita–Avocado Lettuce Wraps
Ginger-Lentil Salad
Creamy Leek and Cauliflower Soup
Asparagus and Sweet Potato Soup
Chicken Lettuce Wraps with Sweet
Potato Hummus
Cream of Asparagus Soup
Southwest-Style Pot Roast
Baked Cashew Chicken
Roasted Radish and Grilled Chicken
Salad
Long and Slow Eggplant Stew
Smoked Turkey–Vegetable Hash

Dinner

Chicken, Mushroom, and Barley Soup
Chicken Chili Fajita Bowl
Turkey and Veggie Fried Rice
Gingered Shrimp and Veggie Stir-Fry

Turkey Burgers with Sweet Potatoes
Savory Lentil and Veggie Stir-Fry
Cornish Game Hens with Mushroom-
Quinoa Stuffing
Wild Rice and Black Bean Salad
Four-Bean Veggie Chili
Quinoa Salad with Radishes and Black
Beans
Turkey and Bell Pepper Rice

Snacks

Mushroom-Spinach Salad
Sardine and Endive Cups
Smoked Oysters and Cucumbers
Eggplant Hummus with Raw Veggies
Lemony White Bean–Dill Hummus and
Veggies
Oven-Baked Sweet Potato Fries
Kale Chips
Lemon-Dressed Artichokes
Deviled Eggs

Smoothies/Beverages

Avocado Smoothie
Coconut-Cherry Smoothie
Raspberry–Almond Milk Smoothie
Cashew Blackberry Smoothie
Beet and Kale Smoothie
Iced Coffee Flavored Drink

Dips and Dressings

Pistachio Dressing
Toasted Sesame Dressing
Pesto
Avocado-Lime Dip
Creamy Cashew Dip
Coconut Sour Cream

Desserts

Cacao-Coconut Ice Cream
Coconut Almond Pudding
Chocolate-Coated Cherries
Blackberry Sorbet
Cacao Cookies

Cashew-Quinoa Hot Cereal SERVES 1

PREP TIME: 5 minutes ■ **TOTAL TIME:** 5 minutes

½ cup hot cooked quinoa

¼ cup cashews

1 cup blackberries

Ground cinnamon to taste

Stevia to taste

In a small bowl, combine all ingredients. Serve hot with sautéed spinach or any other Phase 3 vegetable.

Avocado and Tomato on Toast SERVES 1

PREP TIME: 2 minutes ■ **TOTAL TIME:** 2 minutes

½ avocado

1 slice sprouted-grain bread, toasted

2 tablespoons diced onion

4 ounces turkey bacon, cooked

3 tomato slices

Sea salt to taste

1 grapefruit

Spread the avocado on the toast and top with onion, tomato, and turkey bacon. Sprinkle with salt to taste. Serve with the grapefruit.

Black Bean and Tomato Toast SERVES 1

PREP TIME: 10 minutes ▪ **TOTAL TIME:** 10 minutes

½ **15-ounce can black beans**

3 **tablespoons olive oil**

¼ **cup minced yellow onion**

½ **teaspoon ground cumin**

½ **teaspoon chili powder**

1 **slice sprouted-grain bread, toasted**

1 **tomato, sliced***

Pinch of sea salt

Drain half the liquid from the black beans. Heat a nonstick pan over medium heat and when hot pour in the olive oil and cook the onion for about 5 minutes or until lightly browned. Reduce the heat to low and add the black beans with the remaining liquid, cumin, and chili powder and stir until warmed through. Spread the bean mixture on the toast and top with the sliced tomato. Season with salt and eat immediately.

*In this recipe, the tomato can count as your Phase 3 fruit.

* Spinach-Mushroom Omelet SERVES 1

PREP TIME: 5 minutes ▪ **TOTAL TIME:** 10 minutes

½ teaspoon grapeseed oil

½ teaspoon coconut aminos

¼ cup diced yellow onion

¼ cup sliced mushrooms

1 cup chopped spinach

1 large egg

2 large egg whites or ⅓ cup liquid egg whites

1 tablespoon almond milk

Sea salt and black pepper to taste

1 grapefruit

1 slice sprouted-grain bread, toasted

Heat a nonstick skillet over medium heat and when hot, pour in the grapeseed oil and cook the coconut aminos, onion, and mushrooms for about 5 minutes or until the onions are lightly browned and the mushrooms begin to soften. Add the spinach and stir well. In a small bowl, whisk the egg, egg whites, and almond milk with a dash of salt and pepper. Pour the egg mixture over the veggies and cook for 2 to 3 minutes until the eggs set. Serve with the grapefruit and a slice of sprouted-grain toast.

TIP: If you prefer egg whites only, make sure you add some additional healthy fat, like diced avocado, to this recipe to unleash burn.

Tomato-Topped Tuna Melt SERVES 1

PREP TIME: 5 minutes ■ **TOTAL TIME:** 5 minutes

- 1 3–3½ ounce can water-packed tuna, drained
- 2 tablespoons safflower mayonnaise
- Pinch of chopped fresh cilantro
- 1 slice sprouted-grain bread, toasted
- 1 slice vegan cheddar cheese
- ¼ cup diced or sliced tomato
- 1 cup chopped peaches, plums, or prickly pears

In a small bowl, mix the tuna, mayonnaise, and cilantro. Spread the tuna mixture on the toast and top with the cheese and tomatoes. Toast in a toaster oven until the cheese softens and serve with 1 cup of the fruit on the side.

TIP: In this recipe the almond cheese counts toward your protein serving.

* Oatmeal-Almond Berry Pancakes SERVES 2 (1 SERVING IS 2 PANCAKES)

PREP TIME: 5 minutes ▪ **TOTAL TIME:** 10 minutes

¾ cup almond milk

½ cup almond flour

½ cup rolled or old-fashioned oats

1 tablespoon birch xylitol

2 tablespoons olive oil

1 teaspoon vanilla extract

1 teaspoon baking powder

½ teaspoon baking soda

½ teaspoon sea salt

1 large egg

2 cups blueberries

Put all the ingredients except the blueberries in a blender and blend until smooth. Heat a lightly oiled griddle or frying pan and pour about ½ cup of batter for each of the 4 pancakes onto the hot pan. Cook for about a minute on each side until lightly browned. Serve 2 pancakes with 1 cup of blueberries on top or on the side, and any Phase 3 veggie.

Breakfast Burrito SERVES 1

PREP TIME: 5 minutes ■ **TOTAL TIME:** 15 minutes

3 ounces ground turkey

2 tablespoons chopped onion

2 tablespoons chopped red bell pepper

1 teaspoon finely chopped garlic

½ teaspoon ground cumin

½ teaspoon paprika

1 large egg

1 sprouted-grain tortilla

½ avocado, sliced

¼ cup salsa

1 cup diced prickly pears

1. Heat a nonstick skillet over medium heat and when hot, sauté the turkey, onion, and bell pepper for about 5 minutes or until nicely browned. Add the garlic, cumin, and paprika and stir well. Remove from the heat.

2. In a small bowl, whisk the egg. Choose another nonstick skillet that is the right size to coat thinly with the egg and heat over medium heat. Pour in the egg and cook undisturbed for 2 to 3 minutes or until done. Slide the egg onto a warmed tortilla and top with the turkey mixture, avocado, salsa, and pears. Roll up and enjoy.

Peach-Coconut Tapioca SERVES 2

PREP TIME: 2 minutes ▪ **TOTAL TIME:** 10 minutes

½ cup small tapioca pearls

¼ teaspoon sea salt

1 cup coconut milk

2 large eggs

½ cup xylitol

½ teaspoon vanilla extract

¼ cup coconut flakes

2 cups diced peaches

Any Phase 3 veggie

1. Combine the tapioca, 1 cup of water, and salt in a pot and let soak for 15 minutes or until most of the water is absorbed. Turn the stove on to low heat and add 1 cup of coconut milk. Cook for 10 minutes and remove from the heat.

2. In a small bowl, whisk together the eggs, xylitol, and vanilla. Stir in 1 tablespoon of the hot tapioca to equalize the temperature between the two mixtures, and then stir the egg mixture into the tapioca until evenly mixed. Add the diced peaches and coconut flakes. Serve warm or refrigerate and serve cold with any Phase 3 veggie.

Raspberry-Studded Oatmeal *SERVES 1*

PREP TIME: 5 minutes ▪ TOTAL TIME: 5 minutes

1 cup chopped baby spinach

⅓ cup rolled or old-fashioned oats

Pinch of sea salt

1 cup frozen raspberries

Stevia to taste

¼ cup sunflower seeds

Bring 1 cup of water to a boil in a pot, add the spinach, oats, and salt and cook for about 5 minutes or until done. Add the raspberries and stir until slightly heated and beginning to soften. Add stevia to taste and spoon the oatmeal into a bowl. Sprinkle with sunflower seeds and enjoy.

Fried Egg with Spinach SERVES 1

PREP TIME: 5 minutes ■ **TOTAL TIME:** 10 minutes

1 tablespoon grapeseed oil

1 large egg

1 large egg white

1 slice sprouted-grain bread, toasted

1 cup chopped spinach

Sea salt to taste

1 grapefruit

Heat the grapeseed oil in a skillet over medium heat and when hot, cook the egg and egg white for 1 to 2 minutes or until done, flipping once. Remove the egg from the skillet and set on top of the slice of toast. Put the spinach in the skillet to warm it, tossing it several times. Add salt to taste and serve the spinach with the toast and egg. Serve with the grapefruit.

Almond Berry * Pancakes

SERVES 2 (1 SERVING IS 2 PANCAKES)

PREP TIME: 5 minutes ▪ **TOTAL TIME:** 10 minutes

1 cup almond flour

2 teaspoons baking powder

1 teaspoon ground cinnamon

1 large egg, beaten

⅓ cup almond milk

2 tablespoons grapeseed oil

1 teaspoon vanilla extract

¼ teaspoon stevia

4 cups blackberries, blueberries, or raspberries

Any Phase 3 veggie

In a large bowl, stir together the flour, baking powder, and cinnamon. In a separate bowl, combine the egg, almond milk, oil, vanilla, and stevia. Add to the dry ingredients and mix until thoroughly combined. Heat a lightly oiled griddle or frying pan and pour about ¼ cup of batter for each pancake onto the hot pan. Cook for 1 to 2 minutes on each side until lightly browned. Continue cooking pancakes until there are 8. Top 2 pancakes with 1 cup of berries and serve with any Phase 3 veggie.

Sprouted-Grain Bagel with Smoked Salmon SERVES 1

PREP TIME: 2 minutes ■ **TOTAL TIME:** 2 minutes

½ sprouted-grain bagel

2 tablespoons safflower mayonnaise

6 ounces smoked salmon (nitrate-free, with no sugar added), sliced

Large handful of spinach

1 thick tomato slice

½ cup sliced cucumber

Any Phase 3 fruit

Toast the bagel. Spread with the safflower mayonnaise. Put the salmon slices, spinach, and tomato slice on top of the bagel and serve with sliced cucumber and a piece of Phase 3 fruit.

Dairy-Free Eggs Benedict SERVES 4

PREP TIME: 30 minutes ▪ **TOTAL TIME:** 45 minutes

HOLLANDAISE SAUCE:

- 2 medium egg yolks
- 1 tablespoon fresh lemon juice
- 3 tablespoons coconut oil, heated to about 95°F.
- ½ teaspoon sea salt
- ⅛ teaspoon paprika

EGGS BENEDICT:

- 2 sprouted-grain English muffins, halved and toasted
- 4 cups baby spinach, steamed
- 4 slices cooked nitrate-free turkey bacon
- 4 poached eggs
- 4 cups blackberries or blueberries

1. To make the hollandaise sauce: Fill a blender jar with boiling water, cover with the lid, and let sit for about 10 minutes to heat up the jar. Drain and thoroughly dry the blender jar. Blend the egg yolks and lemon juice on low speed. Slowly pour the heated coconut oil through the feed tube with the blender still on low speed. Season with salt and paprika.

2. To make the eggs Benedict: Top the English muffin halves with equal amounts of spinach and then with bacon and a poached egg. Top with the hollandaise sauce and serve immediately with 1 cup berries per serving.

TIP: This recipe is definitely great for a special occasion. No one would ever believe this dish fits on a "diet."

TIP: The sauce can be made ahead and refrigerated; reheat slowly on low heat, stirring constantly. This sauce is also great as a dipping sauce for veggies.

Artichoke Salad with Avocado and Hearts of Palm SERVES 1

PREP TIME: 5 minutes ■ **TOTAL TIME:** 5 minutes

½ avocado, diced

¼ 14-ounce can hearts of palm, drained and diced

1 6.5-ounce can artichoke hearts, drained and sliced into fourths

1 cup diced tomato*

¼ cup diced red onion

2 tablespoons coconut vinegar

½ teaspoon stevia

½ teaspoon chopped fresh cilantro

¼ teaspoon sea salt

⅛ teaspoon black pepper

2 cups arugula

4 ounces turkey deli meat, sliced into strips

Put all the ingredients except the arugula in a mixing bowl and toss to mix. Serve over a bed of arugula.

*In this recipe the tomato can count as your Phase 3 fruit.

Crab Salad SERVES 1

PREP TIME: 5 minutes ■ **TOTAL TIME:** 5 minutes

2 3–3¾-ounce cans crabmeat

½ cup diced red bell pepper

½ cup shredded red cabbage

¼ cup diced red onion

Juice of ½ lemon (2 tablespoons)

3 tablespoons safflower mayonnaise

Crushed red pepper flakes to taste

2 cups spinach or other Phase 3 greens

1 cup chopped peaches, plums, or other Phase 3 fruit

In a medium mixing bowl, stir together the crabmeat, bell pepper, cabbage, onion, and lemon juice. Add the mayonnaise and mix well. Dress with red pepper flakes to taste. Serve over a bed of spinach or other greens, with the fruit mixed in or on the side.

Avocado-Turkey Lettuce Wrap SERVES 1

PREP TIME: 3 minutes ▪ **TOTAL TIME:** 10 minutes

4 ounces ground turkey

½ cup diced sweet potato

1 teaspoon chopped fresh parsley

Pinch of sea salt

⅛ teaspoon black pepper

6 romaine lettuce leaves

½ avocado, diced

½ cup salsa

1 cup any Phase 3 fruit

Heat a skillet over medium heat and when hot, cook the turkey, sweet potato, and parsley with the salt and pepper for 5 to 8 minutes or until the turkey is browned and the sweet potato is tender. Put the turkey mixture in the lettuce leaves, top with the avocado and salsa, and fold the lettuce leaves around the filling. Serve with the fruit on the side.

Salmon Salad SERVES 1

PREP TIME: 5 minutes ■ **TOTAL TIME:** 5 minutes

- 2 3-ounce cans salmon, drained and flaked
- 1 cup diced red cherry tomatoes*
- ½ cup diced bell pepper
- ¼ cup diced red onion
- ¼ cup safflower mayonnaise
- Juice of ½ lemon (2 tablespoons)
- ½ teaspoon fresh dill weed

Put all ingredients in a small serving bowl and toss to mix.

*In this recipe the tomato can count as your Phase 3 fruit.

TIP: Remember, since veggies are unlimited, don't hesitate to serve this over mixed greens, or in an endive cup or half a bell pepper.

Slow-Cooked Chicken Curry SERVES 4

PREP TIME: 10 minutes ■ **TOTAL TIME:** 3 to 8 hours (slow cooker)

- 1 pound boneless, skinless chicken breasts, cut into 1-inch pieces
- 2 cups sliced red or yellow bell peppers
- ½ cup chopped green onions (scallions), white and green parts
- 3 garlic cloves, chopped
- 2 teaspoons coconut oil
- 2 teaspoons curry powder
- 1 teaspoon minced ginger
- 1 teaspoon chopped fresh parsley
- ½ teaspoon sea salt
- ½ cup coconut milk
- ½ cup organic chicken broth
- ½ cup shredded coconut
- ½ teaspoon stevia
- ⅛ teaspoon turmeric
- 4 cups any Phase 3 fruit

Put all ingredients except the fruit into a slow cooker or Crock-Pot, stir, and cook for 3 to 4 hours on high or 7 to 8 hours on low. Serve with 1 cup of the Phase 3 fruit.

Coconut Chicken with Butternut Squash SERVES 4

PREP TIME: 5 minutes ■ **TOTAL TIME:** 3 to 8 hours (slow cooker)

1 pound whole boneless, skinless chicken breasts

1 cup butternut squash, peeled and cut into 1-inch cubes

1 cup canned coconut milk

3 medium sweet potatoes, peeled and sliced

¼ cup olive oil

2 tablespoons cinnamon

1 teaspoon sea salt

⅛ teaspoon cumin

Any Phase 3 fruit

Put all ingredients except the fruit into a slow cooker or Crock-Pot and cook for 3 to 4 hours on high or 7 to 8 hours on low. Serve with the fruit.

* Shrimp and Avocado Salad SERVES 1

PREP TIME: 5 minutes ■ **TOTAL TIME:** 5 minutes

½ **14-ounce can hearts of palm, drained and diced**

½ **avocado, diced**

¾ **cup cooked shrimp**

¼ **cup diced red onion**

½ **teaspoon chopped fresh cilantro**

2 **tablespoons coconut vinegar**

½ **teaspoon stevia**

¼ **teaspoon sea salt**

⅛ **teaspoon black pepper**

1 **cup arugula**

1 **cup blackberries, blueberries, raspberries, or other Phase 3 fruit**

In a medium mixing bowl, mix together the hearts of palm, avocado, shrimp, onion, and cilantro. Drizzle with vinegar and season with stevia, salt, and pepper. Toss gently to mix well and serve over a bed of arugula, with fruit mixed in or on the side.

Steak Fajita–Avocado Lettuce Wraps *

SERVES 4

PREP TIME: 15 minutes ■ **TOTAL TIME:** 25 minutes

2 tablespoons olive oil

1 pound skirt steak, sliced into ½-inch strips

1 red bell pepper, seeded and thinly sliced

1 yellow bell pepper, seeded and thinly sliced

1 Vidalia onion, thinly sliced

1 cup sliced mushrooms

4 garlic cloves, minced

1 teaspoon chopped chipotle pepper

1 teaspoon chopped fresh cilantro

1 teaspoon crushed red pepper flakes

3 tablespoons lime juice

Head of lettuce, large leaves removed for 4 cups

2 cups diced tomatoes*

1 avocado, diced

Additional ½ serving any Phase 3 fruit

Heat a skillet over medium heat and when hot, heat the olive oil and sear the steak, stirring often, for about 5 minutes or until lightly browned. Add the bell peppers, onion, mushrooms, garlic, chipotle pepper, cilantro, red pepper flakes, and lime juice. Cook, stirring often, for about 5 minutes more or until the vegetables are tender and the steak is cooked to the desired degree of doneness. Spoon the steak mixture into the lettuce cups. Top with equal amounts of diced tomatoes and avocado. Serve with an additional half serving of Phase 3 fruit

*In this recipe the tomato counts as your Phase 3 fruit.

Ginger-Lentil Salad SERVES 4

PREP TIME: 5 minutes ■ **TOTAL TIME:** 5 minutes

2 cups cooked lentils

1 cup diced cucumber

1 cup shredded red cabbage

½ cup diced celery

½ cup minced red onion

3 tablespoons grapeseed oil

2 tablespoons coconut vinegar

1 tablespoon minced ginger

1 tablespoon tamari

4½ teaspoons lemon juice

⅛ teaspoon stevia

⅛ teaspoon turmeric

Pinch of curry powder

½ cup raw sunflower seeds

4 cups diced peaches, plums, prickly pears, or other Phase 3 fruit

In a medium mixing bowl, mix together all ingredients except the sunflower seeds and fruit. Toss well, sprinkle sunflower seeds on top and serve with 1 cup of the fruit on the side per serving.

Creamy Leek and Cauliflower Soup SERVES 6

PREP TIME: 15 minutes ■ **TOTAL TIME:** 45 minutes

2 cups chopped cauliflower

1 cup chopped leeks

1 cup chopped yellow squash

5 garlic cloves, minced

½ cup chopped kale (ribs removed)

2 15-ounce cans garbanzo beans

1 tablespoon olive oil

2 tablespoons tamari

½ teaspoon fresh or dried sage

½ teaspoon chopped fresh parsley

½ teaspoon chopped fresh basil

½ teaspoon sea salt

Pinch of chopped fresh thyme

Pinch of chopped fresh rosemary leaves

1 cup coconut milk

1 heaping tablespoon tahini

6 pieces of any Phase 3 fruit

Put all the ingredients except the tahini and fruit in a large pot. Add 4 cups of water and bring to a boil over high heat. Reduce the heat and simmer for about 20 minutes or until the vegetables are soft. Remove from the heat and stir in the tahini. Let the soup cool and then purée until smooth. You may have to do this in batches. Serve chilled or reheated with 1 piece of Phase 3 fruit.

Asparagus and Sweet Potato Soup SERVES 6

PREP TIME: 10 minutes ▮ **TOTAL TIME:** 45 minutes

2 tablespoons sesame oil

6 cups diced asparagus spears

2 cups diced onions

2 cups diced celery

4 cups organic vegetable broth

2 15-ounce cans white or cannellini beans, drained

1 cup diced cooked sweet potatoes

5 tablespoons chopped fresh parsley

2 teaspoons sea salt

⅓ cup hemp seeds

6 cups of any Phase 3 fruit

Heat the oil in a deep, heavy-bottomed skillet over medium heat and when hot, cook the asparagus, onions, and celery, stirring often for about 5 minutes, until lightly browned. Add the broth, beans, sweet potatoes, parsley, and salt. Bring to a boil and then reduce the heat and simmer for about 30 minutes until the potatoes are tender. Sprinkle a tablespoon of hemp seeds on top of each serving and serve with 1 cup of Phase 3 fruit.

Chicken Lettuce Wraps with Sweet Potato Hummus SERVES 4

PREP TIME: 5 minutes ▪ TOTAL TIME: 30 minutes

1 pound sweet potatoes, peeled and cut into 1-inch pieces

1 15-ounce can garbanzo beans, drained and rinsed

¼ cup fresh lemon juice

¼ cup raw tahini

2 tablespoons olive oil

2 teaspoons ground cumin

1 garlic clove

Sea salt and black pepper to taste

Head of romaine lettuce, large leaves removed for cups

1 pound boneless, skinless chicken breast, cooked and shredded

4 cups chopped tomatoes

1. Fill the bottom of a steamer with water. Place the sweet potatoes in the top part of the steamer, bring to a boil, reduce to a simmer, and cover tightly. Cook the potatoes for about 20 minutes, or until tender. Transfer the sweet potatoes, beans, lemon juice, tahini, olive oil, cumin, garlic, salt, and pepper to a blender. Add 1½ cups of water and purée for about 1 minute, until smooth. Add more water if too thick to spread.

2. Put the lettuce cups on a plate. Spread about ⅓ cup of the hummus on each leaf and top with the chicken and tomatoes. Roll up each lettuce leaf with the filling inside.

TIP: I always try to go organic or at least natural with my chicken because the synthetic estrogens found in poultry not labeled "natural" or "organic" are linked to weight gain and other issues.

TIP: To revisit the whole "is tomato a fruit or vegetable" debate again, feel free to use tomatoes as your fruit in this recipe.

Cream of Asparagus Soup SERVES 4

PREP TIME: 20 minutes ▪ **TOTAL TIME:** 40 minutes

- **4** cups organic chicken or vegetable broth
- **1** medium white or yellow onion, chopped
- **2** garlic cloves, minced
- **2** teaspoons sea salt
- **1** teaspoon black pepper
- **¼** teaspoon ground ginger
- **5** cups chopped asparagus
- **1** 13½-ounce can coconut milk
- **6** ounces nitrate-free deli meat (turkey, chicken, or roast beef)
- **4** pieces of any Phase 3 fruit

In a large pot, bring the broth to a boil over high heat. Add the onion, garlic, salt, pepper, and ginger, reduce the heat, and simmer for 15 minutes, stirring occasionally. Once the onion appears transparent, add the asparagus; it will turn a very bright green in seconds, and 45 seconds after it's added (set a timer if you can), remove the pot from the heat. In a blender, purée the soup in batches until smooth. Return the soup to the pot, stir in the coconut milk and cook until completely incorporated. Add salt to taste. Serve hot or cold with deli meat and a piece of Phase 3 fruit.

Southwest-Style Pot Roast *

SERVES 10

PREP TIME: 10 minutes ▪ **TOTAL TIME:** 3 to 8 hours (slow cooker)

- 1 lean beef roast, about 2½ pounds
- 3 cups seeded and diced bell peppers
- 3 4-ounce cans mild green chiles
- 3 cups sliced mushrooms
- ¼ cup sliced red onion
- 1 tablespoon crushed red pepper flakes
- 1 tablespoon sea salt
- 2 quarts organic beef broth

Put all ingredients into a slow cooker or Crock-Pot and cook for 3 to 4 hours on high or 7 to 8 hours on low.

TIP: This is amazing to shred and place over a bed of lettuce for lunch the next day with chipotle dressing and lime juice.

Baked Cashew Chicken SERVES 4

PREP TIME: 5 minutes ■ **TOTAL TIME:** 45 minutes

1 pound boneless, skinless chicken breasts

½ cup ground cashews

2 tablespoons diced red onion

1 tablespoon coconut oil

1 tablespoon cashew butter

1 teaspoon fresh lemon juice

1 teaspoon sea salt

1 teaspoon chopped fresh cilantro

1 teaspoon fresh thyme leaves

¼ teaspoon paprika

Pinch of crushed red pepper flakes

4 cups blackberries, blueberries, or other Phase 3 fruit

1. Preheat the oven to 375°F.

2. Put chicken breasts in an oven-safe baking dish large enough to hold the breasts in a single layer. In a small bowl, combine the remaining ingredients except the berries and spread over the chicken. Cover with aluminum foil and bake for 30 to 40 minutes or until the chicken is cooked through. Serve with 1 cup of berries per serving.

Roasted Radish and Grilled Chicken Salad SERVES 6

PREP TIME: 10 minutes ■ TOTAL TIME: 1 hour

1½ pounds boneless, skinless chicken breasts

Sea salt and black pepper

1½ pounds trimmed radishes (any type or a mixture)

3 tablespoons olive oil

¼ cup apple cider vinegar

3 green onions (scallions), thinly sliced, white and green parts

2 tablespoons chopped fresh parsley

2 tablespoons chopped fresh dill weed

1 teaspoon sugar-free Dijon mustard or sugar-free yellow mustard

¼ cup safflower mayonnaise

Juice of ½ lemon

6 cups of any Phase 3 fruit

1. Pound chicken breasts into an even thickness and season with salt and pepper. Grill the chicken for about 4 minutes on each side until cooked through. Let the chicken cool and then cut into strips or cubes.

2. Preheat oven to 425°F. Set a large baking sheet in the oven to heat it up.

3. Slice the larger radishes in half and then transfer all the radishes to a mixing bowl and add 2 tablespoons of the olive oil. Toss to coat. Spread the radishes on the hot baking sheet and roast for 25 to 30 minutes, stirring once, until the radishes are tender but not mushy, and are beginning to brown. Watch carefully to prevent overcooking.

4. Meanwhile, in a small bowl, whisk the remaining tablespoon of oil with the vinegar, green onions, herbs, mustard, mayonnaise, and lemon juice. When the radishes are done, allow them to cool slightly and then toss with the vinaigrette. Add salt and pepper to taste. Add the grilled chicken, stir to mix, and serve warm or chilled with 1 cup of the fruit.

Long and Slow Eggplant Stew SERVES 4

PREP TIME: 10 minutes ■ **TOTAL TIME:** 3 to 8 hours (slow cooker)

1 medium eggplant, peeled and diced

2 15-ounce cans garbanzo beans

1 6-ounce can tomato paste

3 cups diced tomatoes

1 cup chopped cauliflower

½ cup diced red onion

½ cup organic vegetable broth

¼ cup coconut vinegar

2 garlic cloves, minced

2 tablespoons lemon juice

1 tablespoon birch xylitol

1 teaspoon celery seed

1 teaspoon sea salt

1 teaspoon fresh or dried oregano

1 teaspoon fresh or dried basil

½ teaspoon crushed red pepper flakes

1 avocado, peeled and diced

4 cups Phase 3 fruit

Put all the ingredients except the avocado and fruit into a slow cooker or Crock-Pot and cook for 3 to 4 hours on high or 6 to 8 hours on low. Serve topped with equal amounts of diced avocado and serve with a cup of Phase 3 fruit.

Smoked Turkey–Vegetable Hash SERVES 4

PREP TIME: 10 minutes ■ TOTAL TIME: 25 minutes

3 tablespoons olive oil	8 cups sliced beet greens
3 large garlic cloves, minced	1½ teaspoons sea salt
¾ cup finely chopped garlic scapes (optional)	1 teaspoon black pepper
4 thick slices smoked turkey, diced	½ cup crushed pecans, walnuts, or pine nuts
1 medium head cauliflower, chopped	4 cups Phase 3 fruit

1. Heat a heavy-bottomed skillet over medium-high heat and when hot, heat 2 tablespoons of the olive oil and cook the garlic for a few seconds until it sizzles. Add the garlic scapes, if using, and the turkey and cook, stirring often for about 5 minutes. Add the cauliflower and cook for 5 minutes more. Add the beet greens and cook, stirring often, for 3 to 5 minutes more, until tender. Add the salt and pepper to the hash and stir to mix.

2. In a small pan on low heat, toast the nuts in the remaining 1 tablespoon of olive oil for about 5 minutes, until they just start to brown. Shake the pan a few times during toasting. Serve the hash topped with the toasted nuts and a cup of the Phase 3 fruit.

Chicken, Mushroom, and Barley Soup SERVES 10

PREP TIME: 10 minutes ■ **TOTAL TIME:** 4 hours

2½ pounds boneless, skinless chicken breasts, diced

2 quarts organic chicken broth

4 cups sliced button or golden mushrooms

2 cups cubed sweet potatoes

1 cup uncooked barley (optional)

1 cup diced yellow onion

¼ cup diced celery

¼ cup tamari

1 fresh or dried bay leaf

1 teaspoon fresh thyme leaves

1 teaspoon dry mustard

½ teaspoon celery seed

2 tablespoons white pepper

5 avocados, diced

Sea salt to taste

Put all ingredients except the avocados and salt in a large pot. Add 2 quarts of water and bring to a boil over high heat. Reduce the heat and let the soup simmer for 4 hours. Before serving, remove the bay leaf, top with diced avocado, and add salt to taste.

TIP: Remember this isn't gluten free, so if you can't eat gluten, don't hesitate to swap the barley with wild rice.

Chicken Chili Fajita Bowl SERVES 4

PREP TIME: 10 minutes ▪ TOTAL TIME: 20 minutes

- 2 tablespoons coconut oil
- 1 pound boneless, skinless chicken breasts, cut into bite-size pieces
- 1 bell pepper, seeded and cut into long, thin strips
- 1 medium white onion, sliced
- ¼ to ½ teaspoon mild chili powder, or to taste
- ¼ teaspoon sea salt, or to taste
- 2 tablespoons coconut aminos
- 2 cups cooked wild rice (optional)
- 2 avocados, diced

Heat a heavy-bottomed skillet over medium heat and when hot, heat the coconut oil and sauté the chicken, stirring often, for about 5 minutes, until lightly browned. Add the bell pepper, onion, chili powder, salt, and coconut aminos. Stir well and cook for about 5 minutes more, until the onion is soft and the chicken is cooked through. Serve over wild rice, if using, and top with avocado.

Turkey and Veggie Fried Rice SERVES 4

PREP TIME: 10 minutes ■ **TOTAL TIME:** 30 minutes

1 pound turkey sausage

¼ cup olive oil

1½ cups julienned carrots

1½ cups diced celery

1½ cups any other sliced Phase 3 vegetables (mushrooms, green onions, jicama, cauliflower)

1 teaspoon sea salt, or to taste

2 cups cooked wild rice (this recipe works best if the rice is left over or cooked the day before)

1. Heat a heavy-bottomed skillet over medium heat and when hot, cook the sausage for about 5 minutes, stirring to break it up, until browned. Transfer the meat to a large mixing bowl.

2. Using the same pan, heat 2 tablespoons of the olive oil and cook the carrots, celery, and other vegetables for about 3 minutes, stirring often. Add ¼ to ⅓ cup of water and salt to taste. Bring to a boil over medium-high heat, reduce the heat and simmer, covered, for about 5 minutes or until the vegetables are tender. Put the vegetables on top of the meat in the bowl.

3. Heat the same skillet over medium heat and when hot, heat the remaining 2 tablespoons olive oil. Add the rice and cook, stirring occasionally, for 8 to 10 minutes, until the rice is browned. Toss the rice with the vegetable-and-meat mixture, taste and add additional salt if necessary, and serve hot.

Gingered Shrimp and Veggie Stir-Fry SERVES 8

PREP TIME: 15 minutes ■ **TOTAL TIME:** 30 minutes

- 4 tablespoons grapeseed oil
- 2 pounds shrimp, cleaned and deveined
- 2 yellow squash, sliced
- 1 cup mushrooms, sliced
- 1 cup chopped bok choy
- ¼ cup sliced asparagus
- 1 cup diced tomatoes
- ¼ cup coconut aminos
- ¼ cup minced ginger
- ½ cup toasted sesame seeds
- 1 tablespoon sea salt herb mix
- 1½ teaspoons crushed red pepper flakes
- 4 cups cooked wild rice

Heat a large heavy-bottomed skillet or wok over medium heat and when hot, heat 1 tablespoon of the oil, tipping the pan to coat it. Add the shrimp and stir-fry for about 4 minutes or until pink. Remove from the pan and set aside. Recoat the pan with the remaining oil and add the squash, mushrooms, bok choy, and asparagus. Stir-fry for about 5 minutes, until the vegetables are slightly tender. Add the tomatoes, coconut aminos, ginger, sesame seeds, salt mix, and red pepper flakes. Cook, stirring often, for 3 minutes. Return the shrimp to the pan, mix with the other ingredients, and cook just until everything is heated through. Serve over rice.

TIP: This meal freezes really well, so if you think you might eat it as a Phase 3 lunch, leave out the wild rice since there are no grains in Phase 3 lunch.

Turkey Burgers with Sweet Potatoes SERVES 4

PREP TIME: 10 minutes ▪ **TOTAL TIME:** 1 hour 20 minutes

4 medium sweet potatoes

2 garlic cloves

½ cup roughly chopped white onion

1 pound lean ground turkey

2 large egg whites or ⅓ cup liquid egg whites

½ cup sprouted-grain bread crumbs

2 teaspoons sea salt

½ teaspoon black pepper

1. Preheat the oven to 400°F. Put the sweet potatoes on the middle rack and bake for 45 minutes to 1 hour or until tender when pierced with a fork.

2. In a blender, purée the garlic and onion. Put the turkey in a large mixing bowl, add the onion mixture, egg whites, bread crumbs, salt, and pepper and mix well. Divide the mixture into four equal portions and then form each portion into a burger.

3. Grill the burgers on an outdoor grill or stovetop grill pan set over high heat for 4 to 5 minutes on each side or until cooked through. Serve with the baked sweet potatoes.

TIP: Make sure to enjoy these with a healthy fat, such as sliced avocado or hummus.

Savory Lentil and Veggie Stir-Fry **SERVES 8**

PREP TIME: 10 minutes ■ **TOTAL TIME:** 20 minutes

1 tablespoon grapeseed oil	Pinch of fresh rosemary leaves
1 onion, sliced	1 fresh or dried bay leaf
½ cup grated carrots	Pinch of turmeric
½ zucchini, sliced	1 teaspoon sea salt
½ yellow squash, sliced	⅛ teaspoon black pepper
¼ cup tamari	4 cups cooked lentils
Pinch of fresh dill weed	½ medium head bok choy, sliced
Pinch of fresh thyme leaves	½ cup spinach
Pinch of ground coriander	4 cups arugula
Pinch of fresh or dried oregano	2 avocados, sliced

Heat a large heavy-bottomed skillet or wok over medium heat and when hot, heat the oil. Cook the onions, carrots, zucchini, and yellow squash, stirring often, for about 5 minutes, until just tender. Add the tamari, dill, thyme, coriander, oregano, rosemary, bay leaf, turmeric, salt, and pepper and stir well. Add the lentils, bok choy, and spinach and cook, stirring often, for about 5 minutes, until the greens are wilted. Remove the bay leaf, and serve over a bed of arugula and top with the avocado.

TIP: Remember that grains are optional in a Phase 3 dinner. Since lentils are also a starch, this might be a time to skip adding an additional grain.

Cornish Game Hens with Mushroom-Quinoa Stuffing SERVES 4

PREP TIME: 10 minutes ■ **TOTAL TIME:** 1 hour 40 minutes

1 cup quinoa

4 tablespoons coconut butter

¼ cup pine nuts

1 teaspoon sea salt, divided

1 cup minced button mushrooms

4 Cornish game hens, skin on

5 garlic cloves, minced

1 teaspoon black pepper

1. Preheat the oven to 375°F.

2. Rinse the quinoa thoroughly and drain. Bring 2 cups of water to a boil, add the quinoa, reduce the heat to medium-low, stir, cover, and simmer for about 15 minutes. Remove from the heat and let the quinoa sit in the covered pot for 5 minutes. Add the coconut butter, pine nuts, ½ teaspoon of the salt, and the mushrooms and combine with a fork.

3. Set the hens on a baking sheet and rub the outside with the remaining ½ teaspoon of salt and the garlic. Stuff the hens with the quinoa mixture and then sprinkle the birds with pepper. Roast on the middle rack of the oven for about 55 minutes, or until the internal temperature reaches 165°F. on an instant-read thermometer inserted between the breast and the leg and not touching bone. Let the hens rest for 10 minutes before serving.

Wild Rice and Black Bean Salad SERVES 1

PREP TIME: 5 minutes ▪ **TOTAL TIME:** 5 minutes

½ cup cooked wild rice

½ cup canned black beans, drained and rinsed

¼ cup sliced green onions (scallions), white and green parts

1 teaspoon chopped fresh cilantro

¼ cup diced tomatoes

½ cup steamed cauliflower, chopped

2 tablespoons coconut aminos

1 garlic clove, minced

3 tablespoons grapeseed oil

Toss all ingredients together and serve.

✳ Four-Bean Veggie Chili SERVES 8

PREP TIME: 5 minutes ▪ **TOTAL TIME:** 3 to 8 hours (slow cooker)

1 15-ounce can each: kidney, pinto, black, and adzuki beans, drained and rinsed

2 cups lentils, rinsed

2 cups cauliflower

1 cup diced celery

1 cup diced tomatoes

4 zucchinis, chopped

2 cups organic vegetable broth

½ cup chopped fresh cilantro or parsley

2 tablespoons chili powder

4 avocados, diced

Put all ingredients except avocados into a slow cooker or Crock-Pot and cook for 3 to 4 hours on high or 7 to 8 hours on low. Serve topped with diced avocado.

Quinoa Salad with Radishes and Black Beans SERVES 4

PHASE 3

DINNER

PREP TIME: 5 minutes ■ **TOTAL TIME:** 1 hour (including time to chill)

1 teaspoon sea salt

½ teaspoon ground cumin

½ teaspoon black pepper

4½ teaspoons olive oil

2 tablespoons coconut vinegar

1 15-ounce can black beans, drained and rinsed

1 cup chopped cucumber

½ cup thinly sliced radishes

2 cups cooked quinoa

2 cups mixed greens

Any Phase 3 dressing

In a mixing bowl, combine the salt, cumin, and pepper. Add the olive oil and vinegar and mix well. Add the beans, cucumber, and radishes and toss to coat with the vinaigrette. Add the quinoa, mix well, and refrigerate for at least 1 hour or until chilled. Serve chilled on a bed of greens and dress with any Phase 3 dressing.

TIP: I like red quinoa in this salad because it gives it a little more punch, but any quinoa will do.

Turkey and Bell Pepper Rice SERVES 4

PREP TIME: 10 minutes ▪ **TOTAL TIME:** 35 minutes

2 tablespoons olive oil

1 pound ground turkey

4 cloves garlic, minced

4 bell peppers, seeded and sliced

1 large white onion, sliced

2 15-ounce cans tomato sauce

½ teaspoon sea salt

½ teaspoon pepper

2 cups cooked wild rice

⅓ cup tahini

Heat a heavy-bottomed skillet over medium heat, add olive oil, and when hot, cook the turkey and garlic for 2 to 3 minutes, breaking it up as it cooks, until browned. Add the peppers and onion and cook, stirring often, for about 8 to 10 minutes until the vegetables are tender. Add the tomato sauce and salt and pepper and stir well. Stir the cooked rice into the skillet, cook over medium-high heat for 2 to 3 minutes, then reduce the heat to low and simmer for about 15 minutes longer to blend the flavors and heat through. Drizzle with the tahini.

Mushroom-Spinach Salad SERVES 2

PREP TIME: 5 minutes ■ **TOTAL TIME:** 5 minutes

- 4 to 6 cups fresh spinach, torn
- 1 cup sliced mushrooms
- 1 cup cherry tomatoes
- ¼ cup cooked, crumbled turkey bacon
- 2 green onions (scallions), diced, white and green parts

DRESSING:
- 6 tablespoons olive oil

- 2 tablespoons apple cider vinegar
- 1 teaspoon birch xylitol, or to taste
- 1 to 1½ teaspoons dry mustard
- ½ teaspoon celery seed
- ¼ teaspoon sea salt
- Black pepper to taste

In a large bowl, toss the spinach, mushrooms, tomatoes, turkey bacon, and green onions. In a jar with a tight-fitting lid, combine the dressing ingredients and shake well. Pour the dressing over the salad and toss. Serve immediately.

TIP: Even if I'm just cooking for myself, I like to make the double portion. I eat half for my snack and save the other half to add to an egg scramble for the next day's Phase 3 breakfast.

Sardine and Endive Cups SERVES 1

PREP TIME: 2 minutes ■ **TOTAL TIME:** 2 minutes

1 3¾-ounce can sardines, packed in olive oil

2 large endive leaves

½ teaspoon prepared horseradish (optional)

Serve the sardines in the endive leaves and top with horseradish, if using.

Smoked Oysters and Cucumbers SERVES 1

PREP TIME: 2 minutes ■ **TOTAL TIME:** 2 minutes

2 ounces smoked oysters, packed in olive oil

½ cup sliced cucumbers

1 fresh basil leaf (optional)

Serve the oysters on top of the cucumber slices. Garnish with a basil leaf, if using.

Eggplant Hummus with Raw Veggies SERVES 10

PREP TIME: 5 minutes ▪ **TOTAL TIME:** 5 minutes

1 15-ounce can garbanzo beans, with liquid

1 15-ounce can white beans, drained and rinsed

1 medium cooked eggplant, peeled and diced

Juice of 1 lemon (3 tablespoons)

2 garlic cloves

1 cup tahini

2 tablespoons coconut aminos

1 teaspoon chopped fresh parsley

⅛ teaspoon fresh dill weed

⅛ teaspoon sea salt

⅛ teaspoon white pepper

Any raw Phase 3 veggies

Put all ingredients except the Phase 3 veggies in a food processor and purée for about a minute or until smooth. Serve with raw veggies.

Lemony White Bean–Dill Hummus and Veggies SERVES 12

PREP TIME: 5 minutes ▪ **TOTAL TIME:** 5 minutes

1 15-ounce can garbanzo beans, with liquid

1 15-ounce can garbanzo beans, drained and rinsed

1 15-ounce can white beans, drained and rinsed

1 cup fresh lemon juice

1 cup tahini

4½ teaspoons minced garlic

1 tablespoon olive oil

1 teaspoon fresh dill weed

1 teaspoon sea salt

Any raw Phase 3 veggies

Put all ingredients except the Phase 3 veggies in a food processor and purée for about a minute until smooth. Serve with raw veggies.

Oven-Baked Sweet Potato Fries SERVES 1

✱

PREP TIME: 5 minutes ▪ **TOTAL TIME:** 40 to 45 minutes

½ cup cooked, sliced sweet potato

1 tablespoon grapeseed oil

½ teaspoon chopped fresh cilantro

½ teaspoon fresh rosemary leaves

Pinch of sea salt

1. Preheat the oven to 375°F.

2. Spread the sweet potato slices on a baking sheet in a single layer (it's okay if a few overlap a little) and drizzle with grapeseed oil. Sprinkle with cilantro and rosemary. Bake for 25 to 30 minutes or until crisp. Sprinkle with salt.

Kale Chips SERVES 1

PREP TIME: 5 minutes ■ TOTAL TIME: 15 to 20 minutes

Bunch of kale	1 teaspoon sea salt
2 tablespoons olive oil	2 to 3 garlic cloves, thinly sliced (optional)

1. Preheat the oven to 350°F.

2. Line a noninsulated baking sheet with parchment paper. Remove the ribs from the kale and tear the leaves into large but still bite-sized pieces. Wash and thoroughly dry the kale. Spread the kale leaves on the baking sheet, drizzle the kale with olive oil, and sprinkle with salt and garlic, if using. Bake for 10 to 15 minutes, until the edges are brown but not burned.

Lemon-Dressed Artichokes SERVES 2

PREP TIME: 5 minutes ▪ **TOTAL TIME:** 20 minutes

2 artichokes	¼ cup tahini
½ cup fresh lemon juice	1 garlic clove, minced
¼ cup olive oil	1 tablespoon chophouse seasoning

Wash and quarter the artichokes, discarding any tough outside leaves. Boil the artichokes in water until the leaves pull off easily and then drain. Whisk together the lemon juice, olive oil, tahini, garlic, and seasoning. Drizzle over the quartered artichokes.

Deviled Eggs SERVES 3

PREP TIME: 5 minutes ▪ **TOTAL TIME:** 5 minutes

3 large hard-boiled eggs	1 teaspoon prepared mustard
1 tablespoon safflower mayonnaise	Pinch of sea salt

Cut the eggs in half lengthwise. Discard one yolk and put the remaining yolks in a small bowl. Finely mash the yolks with a fork. Add the mayonnaise, mustard, and salt and mix well. Fill the egg white halves with the yolk mixture. If the egg yolk mixture is too dry, add a little more mustard.

Avocado Smoothie SERVES 1

PREP TIME: 5 minutes ■ **TOTAL TIME:** 5 minutes

½ avocado

¾ cup coconut milk

½ cup spinach

1 cup diced peaches

½ cup ice cubes

1 tablespoon birch xylitol

Blend all the ingredients until smooth. Serve immediately.

✱ Coconut-Cherry Smoothie SERVES 1

PREP TIME: 5 minutes ■ **TOTAL TIME:** 5 minutes

1 cup hemp milk

1 cup frozen black cherries

½ cup ice cubes

¼ cup shredded coconut

¼ cup cooked quinoa

1 tablespoon raw almond butter

1 teaspoon stevia

Blend all the ingredients until smooth. Serve immediately.

Raspberry–Almond Milk Smoothie SERVES 1

PREP TIME: 5 minutes ▪ **TOTAL TIME:** 5 minutes

1 cup almond milk

1 cup raspberries

½ cup ice cubes

1 tablespoon almond butter

1 teaspoon stevia

Blend all the ingredients until smooth. Serve immediately.

Cashew Blackberry Smoothie SERVES 1

PREP TIME: 5 minutes ▪ **TOTAL TIME:** 5 minutes

1 cup cashew milk or almond milk

1 cup blackberries

½ cup ice cubes

1 tablespoon cashew butter

1 teaspoon stevia

Blend all the ingredients until smooth. Serve immediately.

Beet and Kale Smoothie SERVES 1

PREP TIME: 5 minutes ■ **TOTAL TIME:** 5 minutes

½ cup torn kale (ribs removed first, before tearing kale leaves)

½ cup spinach

½ cup diced raw beets

½ cup diced carrots

½ cup ice cubes

Juice of 1 lime (2 tablespoons)

1 fresh mint leaf

Blend all the ingredients with 4 ounces of spring water until smooth. Serve immediately.

Iced Coffee–Flavored Drink SERVES 1

PREP TIME: 2 minutes ■ **TOTAL TIME:** 2 minutes

2 teaspoons Pero

1 dropper English toffee stevia

¼ cup almond milk

½ cup ice cubes

Blend all the ingredients until smooth. Serve immediately.

TIP: Pero is a caffeine-free herbal coffee alternative but it is not gluten free because it contains barley. I get it at my local grocery store but you can also find it online.

One serving for all dips and dressings is 2 to 4 tablespoons.

Pistachio Dressing SERVES 1

PREP TIME: 5 minutes ▪ **TOTAL TIME:** 5 minutes

2 tablespoons pistachio butter

2 tablespoons olive oil

1 teaspoon minced garlic

½ teaspoon sea salt

Juice of ½ lemon
(2 tablespoons)

Whisk all ingredients together and serve over any Phase 3 salad, meal, or veggies.

Toasted Sesame Dressing SERVES 1

PREP TIME: 2 minutes ▪ **TOTAL TIME:** 2 minutes

2 tablespoons toasted sesame oil

1 teaspoon minced garlic

½ teaspoon sea salt

½ teaspoon white pepper

Pinch of oregano

Juice of ½ lime (1 tablespoon)

Blend all the ingredients until smooth. Serve over any Phase 3 salad, meal, or veggies.

Pesto SERVES 2 TO 4

PREP TIME: 2 minutes ▪ **TOTAL TIME:** 2 minutes

1 cup fresh basil leaves

⅓ cup pine nuts

¼ cup olive oil

1 tablespoon coconut oil

2 garlic cloves, minced

Blend all the ingredients until smooth. Serve as a spread on any Phase 3 wrap or sandwich, drizzle over any Phase 3 meal, or use as a marinade.

Avocado-Lime Dip SERVES 2

PREP TIME: 2 minutes ▪ **TOTAL TIME:** 2 minutes

½ avocado

Juice of ½ lime (1 tablespoon)

1 teaspoon safflower mayonnaise

1 teaspoon chopped fresh cilantro

Sea salt and black pepper to taste

Blend all the ingredients until smooth. Serve with any Phase 3 veggies.

Creamy Cashew Dip SERVES 2

PREP TIME: 2 minutes ■ **TOTAL TIME:** 2 minutes

Juice of 1 lemon
(3 tablespoons)

2 tablespoons cashew butter

2 tablespoons grapeseed oil

1 tablespoon tamari

½ teaspoon stevia

½ teaspoon crushed red pepper
flakes

Blend all the ingredients until smooth. Serve with any Phase 3 meal or veggies.

Cacao-Coconut Ice Cream SERVES 2

PREP TIME: 2 minutes ■ **TOTAL TIME:** 2 minutes

2 cups ice cubes

½ cup coconut milk

¼ cup birch xylitol

¼ cup coarsely chopped pecans

2 tablespoons unsweetened
cacao powder

Put all ingredients in a blender and blend to the desired consistency. Serve right away. If stored in the freezer, let the mixture stand at room temperature for a few minutes before serving.

TIP: Enjoy as a snack, as this dessert contains healthy fat. Just remember to add a Phase 3 vegetable on the side. You can also eat this after a meal if you do an additional day of exercise.

Coconut Almond Pudding SERVES 6

PREP TIME: 5 minutes ■ **TOTAL TIME:** 15 minutes

2 cups coconut milk

1 cup coconut cream

⅔ cup birch xylitol

¼ cup small tapioca pearls

¼ cup almond flour

¼ teaspoon sea salt

3 large eggs, beaten

1 teaspoon vanilla extract

½ cup shredded coconut

In a large sauce pan, whisk the coconut milk and coconut cream with the xylitol, tapioca, flour, salt, and eggs. Cook over medium heat, whisking constantly, for about 8 minutes, until thick. Remove from the heat, stir in the vanilla, and fold in the shredded coconut. Serve warm or chilled.

TIP: Enjoy as a snack, as this dessert contains healthy fat. Just remember to add a Phase 3 vegetable on the side. You can also eat this after a meal if you do an additional day of exercise.

Chocolate-Coated Cherries SERVES 2

PREP TIME: 2 minutes ■ TOTAL TIME: 2 minutes

¼ cup grapeseed oil

2 tablespoons birch xylitol

3 tablespoons unsweetened cacao powder

1 dropper English toffee stevia

1 cup cherries (fresh or frozen)

In a small saucepan set over low heat, heat the oil, xylitol, cacao powder, and stevia until warm and blended. Add the cherries and stir gently to coat. Turn onto a parchment-lined sheet or plate and let cool.

TIP: Since this dessert does contains fruit, it doesn't count as a snack for this phase, but feel free to eat it as a dessert after lunch if you add a day of exercise.

Blackberry Sorbet SERVES 2

PREP TIME: 2 minutes ■ TOTAL TIME: 2 minutes

2 cups blackberries

2 tablespoons birch xylitol

4 cups ice cubes

Blend the ingredients until smooth. Serve right away.

TIP: Since this dessert does not contain healthy fat, it can't count as a snack for this phase. Feel free to add it as a dessert with lunch if you also add a day of exercise. (This sorbet can't be eaten with dinner because there is no fruit in Phase 3 dinner.)

Cacao Cookies SERVES 3 TO 4

PREP TIME: 2 minutes ▪ **TOTAL TIME:** 30 minutes

4 large egg whites at room temperature

½ teaspoon arrowroot powder

3 tablespoons xylitol

¼ cup unsweetened cacao powder

¼ teaspoon sea salt

¼ cup pecans or walnuts, chopped

1. Preheat oven to 325°F.

2. In a large mixing bowl, using a hand mixer or wire whisk, whip the egg whites and arrowroot until stiff peaks form. In another bowl, whisk together the cacao powder, xylitol, salt, and nuts. Slowly add the dry ingredients into the egg whites, making sure to constantly mix while you add. Line a baking sheet with parchment paper. Drop the batter in 1/4 cup amounts onto the parchment paper-lined baking sheet, leaving about 2 inches between each cookie. Bake for 25 minutes, rotating the baking sheet halfway through. Remove from the oven and let cool on the baking sheet. Eat or store for later.

TIP: Enjoy as a snack, as this dessert contains healthy fat. Just remember to add a Phase 3 vegetable on the side. You can also eat this after a meal if you do an additional day of exercise.

Phase 3 Food List

To modify any of the recipes for this phase of the diet, or to make up your own, you may use any of the foods on the following Phase 3 food list.

VEGETABLES AND SALAD GREENS (fresh, canned, or frozen)

Arrowroot

Artichokes

Arugula

Asparagus

Bean sprouts

Beans: *green, yellow (wax), French (string)*

Beets: *greens, roots*

Bok choy

Brussels sprouts

Cabbage, all types

Carrots

Cauliflower florets

Celery

Chicory (curly endive)

Collard greens

Cucumbers

Eggplant

Endive

Fennel

Green chiles

Green onions

Hearts of palm

Jicama

Kale

Kohlrabi

Leeks

Lettuce (any except iceberg)

Mixed greens

Mushrooms

Okra

Onions

Peppers: *bell, pepperoncini*

Radishes

Rhubarb

Seaweed

Spinach

Spirulina

Sprouts

Sweet potatoes/ yams

Tomatoes, fresh and canned: *round, plum, cherry*

Watercress

Zucchini and winter or yellow summer squash

FRUITS (fresh or frozen)

Blackberries

Blueberries

Cherries

Cranberries

Grapefruit

Lemons

Limes

Peaches

Plums

Prickly pears

Raspberries

ANIMAL PROTEIN

Beef: *filet, steaks, lean ground, roast*

Buffalo meat

Calamari

Chicken: *boneless, skinless dark or white meat, ground*

Clams

Corned beef

Cornish game hens

Crab, lump meat

Deli meats, nitrate-free: *turkey, chicken, roast beef*

Eggs, whole

Game: *pheasant*

Halibut fillet

Herring

Lamb

Liver

Lobster meat

Oysters

Pork: *chops, loin roast*

Rabbit

Salmon, fresh, frozen, or nitrate-free smoked

Sardines, packed in olive oil

Sausage, nitrate-free: *chicken, turkey*

Scallops

Sea bass fillet

Shrimp

Skate

Trout

Tuna, fresh or packed in water or oil

Turkey

Turkey bacon, nitrate-free

VEGETABLE PROTEIN

Chickpeas/garbanzo beans	Dried (or canned) beans: *adzuki, black, butter, cannellini, Great*	*Northern, kidney, lima, navy, pinto, white*	Lentils

GRAINS

Barley, black or white	Oats: *steel-cut, old-fashioned*	Sprouted-grain: *bread, bagels, English muffins, tortillas*	Tapioca
Black rice	Quinoa		Wild rice

BROTHS, HERBS, SPICES, CONDIMENTS, AND SUPPLEMENTS

Almond milk, unsweetened	Horseradish, prepared	Nutritional yeast	*sea salt, Simply Organic seasoning*
Brewer's yeast	Ketchup, no sugar added, no corn syrup	Pickles, no sugar added	Sweeteners: *Stevia, Xylitol (birch only)*
Broths: *beef, chicken, vegetable**		Salsa	
Carob chips	Mustard, prepared, dry	Seasonings: *black and white peppers, celery seeds, chophouse seasoning, cinnamon, chili powder, crushed red pepper flakes, cumin, curry powder, onion salt, paprika, raw cacao powder, turmeric,*	Tomato paste
Cashew milk	Natural seasonings: *Bragg Liquid Aminos, coconut amino acids, tamari*		Tomato sauce, no sugar added
Dried herbs: *all types*			Vanilla or peppermint extract
Fresh herbs: *all types*	Noncaffeinated herbal teas or Pero		Vinegar: *any type (except rice)*
Garlic, fresh			
Ginger, fresh			
Hemp milk, unsweetened			

HEALTHY FATS

Avocados	Hummus	Nuts, raw: *almonds, cashews, hazelnuts, pecans, pine nuts, pistachios, walnuts*	Oils: *coconut, grapeseed, olive, sesame, toasted sesame (Asian)*
Coconut, coconut butter, coconut milk, coconut cream, coconut water	Mayonnaise, safflower olives	Nut/seed butters and pastes, raw	Seeds, raw: *flax, hemp, pumpkin, sesame, sunflower*
		Nut flours	Tahini

*****NOTE:** All broths, if possible, should be free of additives and preservatives.

PART III

Appendices

Quick Guide to Vegetarian and Vegan Recipes 210

Master Food List 213

Sample Meal Maps 218

Blank Meal Maps 228

Quick Guide to Vegetarian and Vegan Recipes

PHASE 1	VEGETARIAN	VEGAN
BREAKFAST		
Creamy Brown Rice Cereal	●	●
Piping Hot Quinoa Cereal	●	●
Cinnamon Peaches on Toast	●	●
Buckwheat Flapjacks with Quick and Easy Blackberry Sauce	●	
Apricot Tapioca	●	
Sweet Potato Pancakes	●	
Spicy Southwest Wild Rice Patties	●	
LUNCH		
Toasted Bagel with Herbed White Bean Spread	●	●
Five-Bean Jicama Salad	●	●
Iced-Cold Gazpacho with Watermelon Chunks	●	●
Black Bean–Arugula Wrap	●	●
Puréed Butternut Squash Soup	●	●
Slow-Cooked Minestrone Soup	●	●
Gingered Carrot-Orange Soup	●	●
DINNER		
Tostada	●	●
Sweet Potato Shepherd's Pie	●	●
Broccoli and Fava Bean Stir-Fry	●	●
Ginger Pumpkin-Leek Soup	●	●
Sweet Potato and Broccoli Sauté	●	●
Vegetable Curry	●	●
Vegetarian Lentil Chili	●	●
SNACKS		
Cinnamon-Dusted Apple	●	●
Papaya with Lime Juice	●	●
Cucumber and Tangerine Salad	●	●
Chili-Kissed Mangos	●	●
Ginger Peaches	●	●
Grapefruit with Cinnamon	●	●
Minty Jicama Fruit Salad	●	●
Watermelon with Mint	●	●
Spicy Pomegranate Seeds	●	●
SMOOTHIES/BEVERAGES		
Quinoa-Pear Smoothie	●	●
Three-Melon Smoothie with Mint	●	●
Green Apple Smoothie	●	●
Tropical Smoothie	●	●
Cantaloupe Smoothie	●	●
DIPS AND DRESSINGS		
Black Bean Cilantro Dip	●	●
Tangerine-Cucumber Dressing	●	●
White Bean-Dill Dip	●	●
Chunky Mango Salsa	●	●
Herbed White Bean Spread	●	●
DESSERTS		
Quick-Baked Apple Crisp	●	●
Mint Grilled Pineapple	●	●
Strawberry-Beet, Orange, or Peach Sorbet	●	●

PHASE 2

BREAKFAST	VEGETARIAN	VEGAN
Hard-Boiled Egg Whites Stuffed with Minced Veggies	●	
Rhubarb Meringue	●	
Egg White and Broccoli Omelet	●	
Tempeh-Mushroom Hash (vegans only)		●
LUNCH		
Edamame Chopped Confetti Salad (vegans only)		●
DINNER		
Edamame and Leek Salad (vegans only)		●
Tempeh Vegetable Stew (vegans only)		●
Portobello Mushrooms and Mustard Greens	●	●
Garden Egg White Scramble	●	
Three-Pepper Egg White Souffle	●	
SNACKS		
Mustard Egg Salad	●	
Salty Edamame (vegans only)		●
Pepperty Tofu Jerky (vegans only)		●
SMOOTHIES/BEVERAGES		
Arnold Palmer	●	●
Lime-Mint Smoothie	●	●
Homemade Lemonade	●	●
Colon Cleanse Smoothie	●	●
Detox Smoothie	●	●
Sun Tea Mojito	●	●
DIPS AND DRESSINGS		
Red Bell Pepper Dressing	●	●
Pepperoncini Dressing	●	●
Lemon Vinaigrette	●	●
Chipotle Dressing	●	●
Fiery Southwestern Dip	●	●
DESSERTS		
Lime Sorbet	●	●
Lemon Meringue	●	
Lemon and Lime Ice Pops	●	●

PHASE 3

BREAKFAST	VEGETARIAN	VEGAN
Cashew-Quinoa Hot Cereal	●	●
Black Bean and Tomato Toast	●	●
Spinach-Mushroom Omelet	●	
Avocado and Tomato on Toast	●	●
Peach-Coconut Tapioca	●	
Raspberry-Studded Oatmeal	●	●
Fried Egg with Spinach	●	

	VEGETARIAN	VEGAN
BREAKFAST		
Almond Berry Pancakes	●	
Oatmeal-Almond Berry Pancakes	●	
LUNCH		
Artichoke Salad with Avocado and Hearts of Palm		●
Ginger-Lentil Salad	●	●
Creamy Leek and Cauliflower Soup	●	●
Asparagus and Sweet Potato Soup	●	●
Long and Slow Eggplant Stew	●	●
DINNER		
Lentil and Veggie Stir-Fry	●	●
Wild Rice and Black Bean Salad	●	●
Veggie Chili	●	●
Quinoa Salad with Radishes and Black Beans	●	●
SNACKS		
Eggplant Hummus with Raw Veggies	●	●
Lemony White Bean–Dill Hummus and Veggies	●	●
Sweet Potato Fries	●	●
Kale Chips	●	●
Lemon-Dressed Artichokes	●	●
Deviled Eggs	●	
SMOOTHIES/BEVERAGES		
Avocado Smoothie	●	●
Coconut-Cherry Smoothie	●	●
Raspberry-Almond Milk Smoothie	●	●
Cashew Blackberry Smoothie	●	●
Beet and Kale Smoothie	●	●
Iced Coffee-Flavored Drink	●	●
DIPS AND DRESSINGS		
Pistachio Dressing	●	●
Toasted Sesame Dressing	●	●
Pesto	●	●
Avocado-Lime Dip	●	●
Creamy Cashew Dip	●	●
DESSERTS		
Blackberry Sorbet	●	●
Coconut Almond Pudding	●	
Chocolate-Coated Cherries	●	●
Cacao Cookies	●	
Cacao-Coconut Ice Cream	●	

Master Food List

This is a master list that includes every food you can eat for every phase. Whenever you need to know if it's okay to eat something within your phase, or if you are just looking for what to buy at the store for your phase, look here. Remember, whenever possible, choose organic.

PHASE 1

VEGETABLES AND SALAD GREENS (fresh, canned, or frozen)

Arrowroot

Arugula

Bamboo shoots

Beans: *green, yellow (wax), French*

Beets

Broccoli florets

Cabbage, all types

Carrots

Celery, including tops

Cucumbers

Eggplant

Green chiles

Green onions

Jicama

Kale

Leeks

Lettuce (any except iceberg)

Mixed greens

Mushrooms

Onions, red and yellow

Parsnips

Peas: *snap, snow*

Peppers: *bell, pepperoncini*

Pumpkin

Radishes

Rutabaga

Spinach

Spirulina

Sprouts

Sweet potatoes/ yams

Tomatoes

Turnips

Zucchini and winter or yellow summer squash

FRUITS (fresh or frozen)

Apples

Apricots

Asian pears

Berries: *blackberries. blueberries, mulberries, raspberries*

Cantaloupe

Cherries

Figs

Grapefruit

Guava

Honeydew melon

Kiwis

Kumquats

Lemons

Limes

Loganberries

Mangos

Oranges

Papaya

Peaches

Pears

Pineapples

Pomegranates

Strawberries

Tangerines

Watermelon

ANIMAL PROTEIN

Beef: *filet, lean ground*

Buffalo meat, ground

Chicken: *boneless skinless, white meat*

Corned beef

Deli meats, nitrate-free: *turkey, chicken, roast beef*

Eggs, whites only

Game: *partridge, pheasant*

Guinea fowl

Haddock fillet

Halibut: *fillet, steak*

Pollock fillet

Pork: *tenderloin*

Sardines, packed in water

Sausages, nitrate- free: *turkey, chicken*

Sole fillet

Tuna, fresh or solid white, packed in water

Turkey: *breast meat, lean ground*

Turkey bacon: *nitrate-free*

VEGETABLE PROTEIN

Black-eyed peas

Chana dal/lentils

Chickpeas/ garbanzo beans

Dried or canned beans: *adzuki, black, butter, great northern,* *kidney, lima, navy, pinto, white*

Fava beans, fresh or canned

BROTHS, HERBS, SPICES, CONDIMENTS, AND SUPPLEMENTS

Brewer's yeast

Broths: *beef, chicken, vegetable**

Dried herbs: *all types*

Fresh herbs: *all types*

Garlic, fresh

Ginger, fresh

Horseradish, prepared

Ketchup, no sugar added, no corn syrup

Mustard, prepared, dry

Natural seasonings: *Bragg Liquid Aminos, coconut amino acids, tamari*

Noncaffeinated herbal teas or Pero

Nutritional yeast

Pickles, no sugar added

Salsa

Seasonings: *black and white peppers, cinnamon, chili powder, crushed red pepper flakes, cumin, curry powder, nutmeg, onion salt, raw cacao powder,* *turmeric, sea salt, Simply Organic seasoning*

Sweeteners: *stevia, xylitol (birch only)*

Tomato soup

Tomato paste

Vanilla or peppermint extract

Vinegar: *any type*

GRAINS AND STARCHES

Amaranth

Arrowroot

Barley

Brown rice: *rice, cereal, crackers, flour, pasta, tortillas*

Brown rice cheese or milk

Buckwheat

Kamut

Millet

Oats: *steel-cut, old-fashioned*

Quinoa

Rice milk, plain

Spelt: *pasta, pretzels, tortillas*

Sprouted-grain: *bagels, bread, tortillas*

Tapioca

Teff

Triticale

Wild rice

HEALTHY FATS

None for this phase

PHASE 2

VEGETABLES AND SALAD GREENS (fresh, canned, or frozen)

Arrowroot

Arugula

Asparagus

Beans: *green, yellow (wax), French (string)*

Broccoli florets

Brussels sprouts

Cabbage, all types

Celery

Collard greens

Cucumbers, any type

Endive

Fennel

Green chiles, jalapeños

Green onions

Jicama

Kale

Leeks

Lettuce (any except iceberg)

Mixed greens

Mushrooms

Mustard greens

Onions: *red, white, Vidalia, and yellow*

Peppers: *bell, pepperoncini*

Radishes

Rhubarb

Shallots

Spinach

Spirulina

Swiss chard

Watercress

FRUITS (fresh or frozen)

Lemons

Limes

ANIMAL PROTEIN

Beef, all lean cuts: *filet, tenderloin, strip, sirloin, shell steak, London broil, round steak, rump roast, skirt steak, stew meat, lean ground*

Buffalo meat

Chicken: *boneless, skinless white meat*

Cod/scrod fillet

Corned beef

Deli meats, nitrate-free: *roast beef, chicken, turkey*

Dory fish fillet

Eggs, whites only

Game: *venison, ostrich, elk*

Haddock fillet

Jerky, nitrate-free: *beef, buffalo, turkey, elk, ostrich*

Lamb, lean cuts, ground

Oysters, packed in water

Pork: *loin roast, tenderloin*

Salmon: *nitrate-free smoked*

Sardines, packed in water

Sole fillet

Tuna, packed in water

Turkey: *breast steaks, lean ground*

Turkey bacon: *nitrate-free*

VEGETABLE PROTEIN

None this phase

BROTHS, HERBS, SPICES, CONDIMENTS, AND SUPPLEMENTS

Brewer's yeast

Broths: *beef, chicken, vegetable**

Dried herbs: *all types*

Fresh herbs: *all types*

Garlic, fresh, powdered

Ginger, fresh

Horseradish, prepared

Mustard, prepared, dry

Natural seasonings: *Bragg Liquid Aminos, coconut amino acids, tamari*

Noncaffeinated herbal teas or Pero

Nutrtional yeast

Pickles, no sugar added

Seasonings: *black and white peppers, cayenne, chili powder, chili paste, chipotle, cinnamon, crushed red pepper flakes, cumin, curry powder, lemon pepper, liquid smoke, nutmeg, onion powder, onion salt, paprika, raw cacao powder, sea salt*

Sweeteners: *stevia, xylitol (birch only)*

Tabasco

Vanilla or peppermint extract

Vinegar, any type (except rice)

GRAINS AND STARCHES

None this phase

HEALTHY FATS

None this phase

*NOTE: All broths, if possible, should be free of additives and preservatives.

PHASE 3

VEGETABLES AND SALAD GREENS (fresh, canned, or frozen)

Arrowroot

Artichokes

Arugula

Asparagus

Bean sprouts

Beans: *green, yellow (wax), French (string)*

Beets: *greens, roots*

Bok choy

Broccoli

Brussels sprouts

Cabbage, all types

Carrots

Cauliflower florets

Celery

Chicory (curly endive)

Collard greens

Cucumbers

Eggplant

Endive

Fennel

Green chiles

Green onions

Hearts of palm

Jicama

Kale

Kohlrabi

Leeks

Lettuce (any except iceberg)

Mixed greens

Mushrooms

Okra

Olives, any type

Onions

Peppers: *bell, pepperoncini*

Radishes

Rhubarb

Seaweed

Spinach

Spirulina

Sprouts

Sweet potatoes/yams

Tomatoes, fresh and canned: *round, plum, cherry*

Watercress

Zucchini and winter or yellow summer squash

FRUITS (fresh or frozen)

Blackberries

Blueberries

Cherries

Cranberries

Grapefruit

Lemons

Limes

Peaches

Plums

Prickly pears

Raspberries

ANIMAL PROTEIN

Beef: *filet, steaks, lean ground, roast*

Buffalo meat

Calamari

Chicken: *boneless, skinless dark or white meat, ground*

Clams

Corned beef

Cornish game hens

Crab, lump meat

Deli meats, nitrate-free: *turkey, chicken, roast beef*

Eggs, whole

Game: *pheasant*

Halibut fillet

Herring

Lamb

Liver

Lobster meat

Oysters

Pork: *chops, loin roast*

Rabbit

Salmon, fresh, frozen, or nitrate-free smoked

Sardines, packed in olive oil

Sausage, nitrate-free: *chicken, turkey*

Scallops

Sea bass fillet

Shrimp

Skate

Trout

Tuna, fresh or packed in water or oil

Turkey

Turkey bacon, nitrate-free

VEGETABLE PROTEIN

Almond flour

Chickpeas/garbanzo beans

Dried (or canned) beans: *adzuki, black, butter, cannellini, Great Northern, kidney, lima, navy, pinto, white*

Lentils

Vegan cheddar cheese

GRAINS

Barley, black or white

Black rice

Oats: *steel-cut, old-fashioned*

Quinoa

Sprouted-grain: *bread, bagels, English muffins, tortillas*

Tapioca

Wild rice

BROTHS, HERBS, SPICES, CONDIMENTS, AND SUPPLEMENTS

Almond milk, unsweetned

Brewer's yeast

Broths: *beef, chicken, vegetable**

Carob chips

Cashew milk

Dried herbs: *all types*

Fresh herbs: *all types*

Garlic, fresh

Ginger, fresh

Hemp milk, unsweetened

Horseradish, prepared

Ketchup, no sugar added, no corn syrup

Mustard, prepared, dry

Natural seasonings: *Bragg Liquid Aminos, coconut amino acids, tamari*

Noncaffeinated herbal teas or Pero

Nutrtional yeast

Pickles, no sugar added

Salsa

Seasonings: *black and white peppers, celery seed, chophouse seasoning, cinnamon, chili powder, crushed red pepper flakes, cumin, curry powder, onion salt, paprika, raw cacao powder, turmeric,*

sea salt, Simply Organic seasoning

Sweeteners: *Stevia, Xylitol (birch only)*

Tomato paste

Tomato sauce, no sugar added

Vanilla or peppermint extract

Vinegar: *any type (except rice)*

HEALTHY FATS

Avocados

Coconut, coconut butter, coconut milk, coconut cream, coconut water

Hummus

Mayonnaise, safflower

Nuts, raw: *almonds, cashews, hazelnuts, pecans, pine nuts, pistachios, walnuts*

Nut/seed butters and pastes, raw

Nut flours

Oils: *coconut, grapeseed, olive, sesame, toasted sesame (Asian)*

Seeds, raw: *flax, hemp, pumpkin, sesame, sunflower*

Tahini

Sample Meal Maps

WEEK ONE MEAL MAP

	BREAKFAST	SNACK	LUNCH	SNACK	DINNER	EXERCISE	WATER	
__:___am/pm **WAKE TIME** **Monday** _____ **WEIGHT**	__:___am/pm P1 creamy brown rice cereal with fruit	__:___am/pm P1 fruit salad	__:___am/pm P1 tangy tuna and veggie melt	__:___am/pm P1 cucumber and tangerine salad	__:___am/pm P1 pasta and simmered tomato-meat sauce			PHASE 1: UNWIND STRESS
__:___am/pm **WAKE TIME** **Tuesday** _____ **WEIGHT**	__:___am/pm P1 buckwheat flapjacks	__:___am/pm P1 watermelon with mint	__:___am/pm P1 spinach salad with seared pork and squash	__:___am/pm P1 orange sorbet	__:___am/pm P1 vegetable curry			
__:___am/pm **WAKE TIME** **Wednesday** _____ **WEIGHT**	__:___am/pm P2 spinach and mushroom scramble	__:___am/pm P2 smoked salmon and celery	__:___am/pm P2 tuna salad in endive leaves	__:___am/pm P2 mustard egg salad	__:___am/pm P2 rosemary pork tenderloin with mustard greens			PHASE 2: UNLOCK FAT STORES
__:___am/pm **WAKE TIME** **Thursday** _____ **WEIGHT**	__:___am/pm P2 jicama with bacon and lime	__:___am/pm P2 smoked salmon and and cucumbers	__:___am/pm P2 buffalo tip salad	__:___am/pm P2 roast beef-wrapped pickles	__:___am/pm P2 turkey meat loaf and asparagus			

	BREAKFAST	SNACK	LUNCH	SNACK	DINNER	EXERCISE	WATER
__:__ am/pm **WAKE TIME** **Friday** _____ **WEIGHT**	__:__ am/pm P3 spinach-mushroom omelet	__:__ am/pm P3 eggplant hummus and raw veggies	__:__ am/pm P3 cream of asparagus soup	__:__ am/pm ¼ cup pine nuts	__:__ am/pm P3 savory lentil and veggie stir-fry		
__:__ am/pm **WAKE TIME** **Saturday** _____ **WEIGHT**	__:__ am/pm P3 avocado smoothie	__:__ am/pm P3 kale chips	__:__ am/pm P3 artichoke salad with avocado and hearts of palm	__:__ am/pm P3 deviled eggs	__:__ am/pm P3 turkey and veggie fried rice		
__:__ am/pm **WAKE TIME** **Sunday** _____ **WEIGHT**	__:__ am/pm P3 raspberry-studded oatmeal	__:__ am/pm P3 lemon-dressed artichokes	__:__ am/pm P3 chicken lettuce wraps with sweet potato hummus	__:__ am/pm P3 oven-baked sweet potato fries	__:__ am/pm P3 chicken, mushroom, and barley soup		

PHASE 3: UNLEASH THE BURN

WEEK TWO MEAL MAP

	BREAKFAST	SNACK	LUNCH	SNACK	DINNER	EXERCISE	WATER	
Monday __:__ am/pm WAKE TIME _____ WEIGHT	P1 cinnamon peaches on toast	1 apple	P1 mediterranean turkey with wild rice	P1 quick baked apple crisp	P1 stuffed cornish game hens			PHASE 1: UNWIND STRESS
Tuesday __:__ am/pm WAKE TIME _____ WEIGHT	P1 piping hot quinoa cereal	1 asian pear	P1 puréed butternut squash soup with a side of mixed greens and mushrooms	P1 papaya with lime juice	P1 slow-cooked corned beef brisket and cabbage			
Wednesday __:__ am/pm WAKE TIME _____ WEIGHT	P2 southwestern breakfast stir-fry	P2 garden meatballs	P2 buffalo wrap	P2 wild sardine pâté	P2 steak fajita lettuce wraps			PHASE 2: UNLOCK FAT STORES
Thursday __:__ am/pm WAKE TIME _____ WEIGHT	P2 rhubarb meringue	P2 steak fajita lettuce wraps	P2 home-style turkey meat loaf and steamed broccoli	P2 garden meatballs	P2 baked cod and veggies			

	BREAKFAST	SNACK	LUNCH	SNACK	DINNER	EXERCISE	WATER	
__:___am/pm **WAKE TIME** **Friday** _____ **WEIGHT**	__:___am/pm P3 fried egg with spinach	__:___am/pm P3 mushroom-spinach salad	__:___am/pm P3 crab salad	__:___am/pm P3 eggplant hummus with cucumbers	__:___am/pm P3 turkey and bell pepper rice and a side of steamed cauliflower			
__:___am/pm **WAKE TIME** **Saturday** _____ **WEIGHT**	__:___am/pm P3 breakfast burrito	__:___am/pm veggies and hummus	__:___am/pm P3 creamy leek and cauliflower soup	__:___am/pm P3 smoked oysters and cucumbers	__:___am/pm P3 four-bean veggie chili			
__:___am/pm **WAKE TIME** **Sunday** _____ **WEIGHT**	__:___am/pm P3 beet and kale smoothie and 1 slice Ezekiel bread with almond butter	__:___am/pm celery with almond butter	__:___am/pm P3 salmon salad	__:___am/pm P3 avocado smoothie	__:___am/pm P3 cornish game hens with mushroom-quinoa stuffing and a side of mixed greens			PHASE 3: UNLEASH THE BURN

WEEK THREE MEAL MAP

	BREAKFAST	SNACK	LUNCH	SNACK	DINNER	EXERCISE	WATER	
__:____am/pm **WAKE TIME** **Monday** _____ **WEIGHT**	__:____am/pm P1 piping hot quinoa cereal	__:____am/pm 1 cup mango	__:____am/pm P1 ice-cold gazpacho with watermelon chunks	__:____am/pm P1 green apple smoothie	__:____am/pm P1 ginger pumpkin-leek soup and a side of sautéed kale			**PHASE 1: UNWIND STRESS**
__:____am/pm **WAKE TIME** **Tuesday** _____ **WEIGHT**	__:____am/pm P1 apricot tapioca	__:____am/pm P1 tropical smoothie	__:____am/pm P1 sloppy joe turkey wrap	__:____am/pm P1 strawberry-beet sorbet	__:____am/pm P1 tostada			
__:____am/pm **WAKE TIME** **Wednesday** _____ **WEIGHT**	__:____am/pm P2 detox smoothie	__:____am/pm P2 summer salsa with turkey bacon chips	__:____am/pm P2 rosemary pork tenderloin with mustard greens	__:____am/pm P2 mustard egg salad	__:____am/pm P2 New York strip steak with broccoli			**PHASE 2: UNLOCK FAT STORES**
__:____am/pm **WAKE TIME** **Thursday** _____ **WEIGHT**	__:____am/pm P2 hard-boiled egg whites stuffed with minced veggies	__:____am/pm P2 New York strip steak with broccoli in lettuce cups	__:____am/pm P2 warm asparagus and bacon salad	__:____am/pm P2 turkey jerky and cucumbers	__:____am/pm P2 lemon mustard pepper chicken			

	BREAKFAST	SNACK	LUNCH	SNACK	DINNER	EXERCISE	WATER
Friday ___:___am/pm WAKE TIME _____ WEIGHT	___:___am/pm P3 cashew-quinoa hot cereal	___:___am/pm ¼ cup raw cashews	___:___am/pm P3 steak fajita—avocado lettuce wrap	___:___am/pm P3 oven-baked sweet potato fries and asparagus spears	___:___am/pm P3 chicken, mushroom, and barley soup and a side of Brussels sprouts		
Saturday ___:___am/pm WAKE TIME _____ WEIGHT	___:___am/pm P3 oatmeal-almond berry pancakes	___:___am/pm veggies and hummus	___:___am/pm P3 chicken lettuce wraps with sweet potato hummus	___:___am/pm P3 lemon-dressed artichokes	___:___am/pm P3 gingered shrimp and veggie stir-fry		
Sunday ___:___am/pm WAKE TIME _____ WEIGHT	___:___am/pm P3 peach-coconut tapioca	___:___am/pm P3 avocado smoothie	___:___am/pm P3 salmon salad	___:___am/pm P3 deviled eggs	___:___am/pm P3 chicken chili fajita bowl		

PHASE 3: UNLEASH THE BURN

WEEK FOUR MEAL MAP

	BREAKFAST	SNACK	LUNCH	SNACK	DINNER	EXERCISE	WATER	
Monday ___:___am/pm WAKE TIME _____ WEIGHT	___:___am/pm P1 piping hot quinoa cereal	___:___am/pm P1 papaya with lime juice	___:___am/pm P1 sloppy joe turkey wrap	___:___am/pm 2 tangerines	___:___am/pm P1 dover sole with tomato and brown rice			PHASE 1: UNWIND STRESS
Tuesday ___:___am/pm WAKE TIME _____ WEIGHT	___:___am/pm P1 spicy southwest wild rice patties	___:___am/pm P1 quick baked apple crisp	___:___am/pm P1 gingered carrot-orange soup	___:___am/pm 1 cup pineapple	___:___am/pm P1 warm steak salad over a bed of spinach			
Wednesday ___:___am/pm WAKE TIME _____ WEIGHT	___:___am/pm P2 spinach and mushroom scramble	___:___am/pm P2 summer salsa with turkey bacon chips	___:___am/pm P2 broiled mustard-coated steak	___:___am/pm P2 garden meatballs	___:___am/pm P2 chicken with shiitake mushrooms and mustard greens			PHASE 2: UNLOCK FAT STORES
Thursday ___:___am/pm WAKE TIME _____ WEIGHT	___:___am/pm P2 steak and eggs	___:___am/pm P2 turkey jerky and cucumbers	___:___am/pm P2 buffalo tip salad	___:___am/pm P2 smoked salmon and cucumbers	___:___am/pm P2 marinated chicken and veggie kabobs			

	BREAKFAST	SNACK	LUNCH	SNACK	DINNER	EXERCISE	WATER
__:___am/pm **WAKE TIME** **Friday** _____ **WEIGHT**	__:___am/pm P3 fried egg with spinach	__:___am/pm P3 coconut-cherry smoothie with radishes	__:___am/pm P3 asparagus and sweet potato soup	__:___am/pm P3 veggies with avocado-lime dip	__:___am/pm P3 quinoa salad with radishes and black beans and a side of sautéed leeks		
__:___am/pm **WAKE TIME** **Saturday** _____ **WEIGHT**	__:___am/pm P3 beet and kale smoothie and 1 slice Ezekiel bread with almond butter	__:___am/pm P3 raspberry–almond milk smoothie and carrot sticks	__:___am/pm P3 ginger-lentil salad	__:___am/pm P3 veggies with avocado-lime dip	__:___am/pm P3 turkey and veggie fried rice		
__:___am/pm **WAKE TIME** **Sunday** _____ **WEIGHT**	__:___am/pm P3 tomato-topped tuna melt	__:___am/pm P3 chocolate-coated cherries	__:___am/pm P3 slow-cooked chicken curry	__:___am/pm P3 sardine and cucumber canapés	__:___am/pm P3 wild rice and black bean salad		

PHASE 3: UNLEASH THE BURN

BONUS VEGETARIAN WEEK:

	BREAKFAST	SNACK	LUNCH	SNACK	DINNER	EXERCISE	WATER	
__:___am/pm **WAKE TIME** **Monday** _____ **WEIGHT**	__:___am/pm P1 creamy brown rice cereal	__:___am/pm P1 cinnamon-dusted apple	__:___am/pm P1 five-bean jicama salad	__:___am/pm P1 ginger peaches	__:___am/pm P1 sweet potato and broccoli sauté			**PHASE 1: UNWIND STRESS**
__:___am/pm **WAKE TIME** **Tuesday** _____ **WEIGHT**	__:___am/pm P1 apricot tapioca	__:___am/pm P1 tropical smoothie	__:___am/pm P1 gingered carrot-orange soup	__:___am/pm P1 watermelon with mint	__:___am/pm P1 tostada with a side of sautéed spinach			
__:___am/pm **WAKE TIME** **Wednesday** _____ **WEIGHT**	__:___am/pm P2 rhubarb meringue	__:___am/pm P2 mustard egg salad	__:___am/pm P2 egg white and broccoli omelet with a side of grilled asparagus	__:___am/pm P2 lemon meringue	__:___am/pm P2 portobello mushrooms and mustard greens			**PHASE 2: UNLOCK FAT STORES**
__:___am/pm **WAKE TIME** **Thursday** _____ **WEIGHT**	__:___am/pm P2 hard-boiled egg whites stuffed with minced veggies	__:___am/pm P2 leftover lettuce cups with dressing	__:___am/pm P2 egg white and broccoli omelet with salad of mixed greens, onions, and mushrooms	__:___am/pm P2 peppery tofu jerky	__:___am/pm P2 garden egg white scramble with a side of sautéed spinach			

	BREAKFAST	SNACK	LUNCH	SNACK	DINNER	EXERCISE	WATER
__:___am/pm **WAKE TIME** **Friday** _____ **WEIGHT**	__:___am/pm P3 peach-coconut tapioca	__:___am/pm P3 eggplant hummus with raw veggies	__:___am/pm P3 artichoke salad with avocado and hearts of palm	__:___am/pm P3 kale chips	__:___am/pm P3 cream of asparagus soup with a side of steamed Brussels sprouts		
__:___am/pm **WAKE TIME** **Saturday** _____ **WEIGHT**	__:___am/pm P3 almond berry pancakes with a side of jicama	__:___am/pm ¼ cup raw almonds and 1 sliced bell pepper	__:___am/pm P3 ginger-lentil salad	__:___am/pm P3 oven-baked sweet potato fries	__:___am/pm P3 four-bean veggie chili		
__:___am/pm **WAKE TIME** **Sunday** _____ **WEIGHT**	__:___am/pm P3 fried egg with spinach	__:___am/pm P3 coconut almond pudding	__:___am/pm P3 asparagus and sweet potato soup	__:___am/pm P3 avocado smoothie	__:___am/pm P3 savory lentil and veggie stir-fry		

PHASE 3: UNLEASH THE BURN

Blank Meal Maps

BLANK MEAL MAP

	BREAKFAST	SNACK	LUNCH	SNACK	DINNER	EXERCISE	WATER	
__:__ am/pm **WAKE TIME** **Monday** _____ **WEIGHT**	__:__ am/pm P1 grain P1 fruit	__:__ am/pm P1 fruit	__:__ am/pm P1 grain P1 protein P1 fruit P1 veggie	__:__ am/pm P1 fruit	__:__ am/pm P1 grain P1 protein P1 veggie			PHASE 1: UNWIND STRESS
__:__ am/pm **WAKE TIME** **Tuesday** _____ **WEIGHT**	__:__ am/pm P1 grain P1 fruit	__:__ am/pm P1 fruit	__:__ am/pm P1 grain P1 protein P1 fruit P1 veggie	__:__ am/pm P1 fruit	__:__ am/pm P1 grain P1 protein P1 veggie			
__:__ am/pm **WAKE TIME** **Wednesday** _____ **WEIGHT**	__:__ am/pm P2 protein P2 veggie	__:__ am/pm P2 protein	__:__ am/pm P2 protein P2 veggie	__:__ am/pm P2 protein	__:__ am/pm P2 protein P2 veggie			PHASE 2: UNLOCK FAT STORES
__:__ am/pm **WAKE TIME** **Thursday** _____ **WEIGHT**	__:__ am/pm P2 protein P2 veggie	__:__ am/pm P2 protein	__:__ am/pm P2 protein P2 veggie	__:__ am/pm P2 protein	__:__ am/pm P2 protein P2 veggie			

	BREAKFAST	SNACK	LUNCH	SNACK	DINNER	EXERCISE	WATER
__:____am/pm **WAKE TIME** **Friday** _____ **WEIGHT**	__:____am/pm P3 fruit P3 healthy fat/protein P3 grain P3 veggie	__:____am/pm P3 veggie P3 healthy fat/protein	__:____am/pm P3 healthy fat/protein P3 veggie P3 fruit	__:____am/pm P3 veggie P3 healthy fat/protein	__:____am/pm P3 healthy fat/protein P3 veggie P3 grain (optional)		
__:____am/pm **WAKE TIME** **Saturday** _____ **WEIGHT**	__:____am/pm P3 fruit P3 healthy fat/protein P3 grain P3 veggie	__:____am/pm P3 veggie P3 healthy fat/protein	__:____am/pm P3 veggie P3 healthy fat/protein P3 fruit	__:____am/pm P3 veggie P3 healthy fat/protein	__:____am/pm P3 healthy fat/protein P3 veggie P3 grain (optional)		
__:____am/pm **WAKE TIME** **Sunday** _____ **WEIGHT**	__:____am/pm P3 fruit P3 healthy fat/protein P3 grain P3 veggie	__:____am/pm P3 veggie P3 healthy fat/protein	__:____am/pm P3 healthy fat/protein P3 veggie P3 fruit	__:____am/pm P3 veggie P3 healthy fat/protein	__:____am/pm P3 healthy fat/protein P3 veggie P3 grain (optional)		

PHASE 3: UNLEASH THE BURN

BLANK MEAL MAP

	BREAKFAST	SNACK	LUNCH	SNACK	DINNER	EXERCISE	WATER	
__:__am/pm **WAKE TIME** **Monday** _____ **WEIGHT**	__:__am/pm P1 grain P1 fruit	__:__am/pm P1 fruit	__:__am/pm P1 grain P1 protein P1 fruit P1 veggie	__:__am/pm P1 fruit	__:__am/pm P1 grain P1 protein P1 veggie			PHASE 1: UNWIND STRESS
__:__am/pm **WAKE TIME** **Tuesday** _____ **WEIGHT**	__:__am/pm P1 grain P1 fruit	__:__am/pm P1 fruit	__:__am/pm P1 grain P1 protein P1 fruit P1 veggie	__:__am/pm P1 fruit	__:__am/pm P1 grain P1 protein P1 veggie			
__:__am/pm **WAKE TIME** **Wednesday** _____ **WEIGHT**	__:__am/pm P2 protein P2 veggie	__:__am/pm P2 protein	__:__am/pm P2 protein P2 veggie	__:__am/pm P2 protein	__:__am/pm P2 protein P2 veggie			PHASE 2: UNLOCK FAT STORES
__:__am/pm **WAKE TIME** **Thursday** _____ **WEIGHT**	__:__am/pm P2 protein P2 veggie	__:__am/pm P2 protein	__:__am/pm P2 protein P2 veggie	__:__am/pm P2 protein	__:__am/pm P2 protein P2 veggie			

	BREAKFAST	SNACK	LUNCH	SNACK	DINNER	EXERCISE	WATER
__:___am/pm **WAKE TIME** **Friday** _____ **WEIGHT**	__:___am/pm P3 fruit P3 healthy fat/protein P3 grain P3 veggie	__:___am/pm P3 veggie P3 healthy fat/protein	__:___am/pm P3 healthy fat/protein P3 veggie P3 fruit	__:___am/pm P3 veggie P3 healthy fat/protein	__:___am/pm P3 healthy fat/protein P3 veggie P3 grain (optional)		
__:___am/pm **WAKE TIME** **Saturday** _____ **WEIGHT**	__:___am/pm P3 fruit P3 healthy fat/protein P3 grain P3 veggie	__:___am/pm P3 veggie P3 healthy fat/protein	__:___am/pm P3 healthy fat/protein P3 veggie P3 fruit	__:___am/pm P3 veggie P3 healthy fat/protein	__:___am/pm P3 healthy fat/protein P3 veggie P3 grain (optional)		
__:___am/pm **WAKE TIME** **Sunday** _____ **WEIGHT**	__:___am/pm P3 fruit P3 healthy fat/protein P3 grain P3 veggie	__:___am/pm P3 veggie P3 healthy fat/protein	__:___am/pm P3 healthy fat/protein P3 veggie P3 fruit	__:___am/pm P3 veggie P3 healthy fat/protein	__:___am/pm P3 healthy fat/protein P3 veggie P3 grain (optional)		

PHASE 3: UNLEASH THE BURN

BLANK MEAL MAP

	BREAKFAST	SNACK	LUNCH	SNACK	DINNER	EXERCISE	WATER	
__:___am/pm **WAKE TIME** **Monday** _____ WEIGHT	__:___am/pm P1 grain P1 fruit	__:___am/pm P1 fruit	__:___am/pm P1 grain P1 protein P1 fruit P1 veggie	__:___am/pm P1 fruit	__:___am/pm P1 grain P1 protein P1 veggie			PHASE 1: UNWIND STRESS
__:___am/pm **WAKE TIME** **Tuesday** _____ WEIGHT	__:___am/pm P1 grain P1 fruit	__:___am/pm P1 fruit	__:___am/pm P1 grain P1 protein P1 fruit P1 veggie	__:___am/pm P1 fruit	__:___am/pm P1 grain P1 protein P1 veggie			
__:___am/pm **WAKE TIME** **Wednesday** _____ WEIGHT	__:___am/pm P2 protein P2 veggie	__:___am/pm P2 protein	__:___am/pm P2 protein P2 veggie	__:___am/pm P2 protein	__:___am/pm P2 protein P2 veggie			PHASE 2: UNLOCK FAT STORES
__:___am/pm **WAKE TIME** **Thursday** _____ WEIGHT	__:___am/pm P2 protein P2 veggie	__:___am/pm P2 protein	__:___am/pm P2 protein P2 veggie	__:___am/pm P2 protein	__:___am/pm P2 protein P2 veggie			

	BREAKFAST	SNACK	LUNCH	SNACK	DINNER	EXERCISE	WATER
__:__ am/pm **WAKE TIME** **Friday** _____ **WEIGHT**	__:__ am/pm P3 fruit P3 healthy fat/protein P3 grain P3 veggie	__:__ am/pm P3 veggie P3 healthy fat/protein	__:__ am/pm P3 healthy fat/protein P3 veggie P3 fruit	__:__ am/pm P3 veggie P3 healthy fat/protein	__:__ am/pm P3 healthy fat/protein P3 veggie P3 grain (optional)		
__:__ am/pm **WAKE TIME** **Saturday** _____ **WEIGHT**	__:__ am/pm P3 fruit P3 healthy fat/protein P3 grain P3 veggie	__:__ am/pm P3 veggie P3 healthy fat/protein	__:__ am/pm P3 healthy fat/protein P3 veggie P3 fruit	__:__ am/pm P3 veggie P3 healthy fat/protein	__:__ am/pm P3 healthy fat/protein P3 veggie P3 grain (optional)		
__:__ am/pm **WAKE TIME** **Sunday** _____ **WEIGHT**	__:__ am/pm P3 fruit P3 healthy fat/protein P3 grain P3 veggie	__:__ am/pm P3 veggie P3 healthy fat/protein	__:__ am/pm P3 healthy fat/protein P3 veggie P3 fruit	__:__ am/pm P3 veggie P3 healthy fat/protein	__:__ am/pm P3 healthy fat/protein P3 veggie P3 grain (optional)		

PHASE 3: UNLEASH THE BURN

BLANK MEAL MAP

	BREAKFAST	SNACK	LUNCH	SNACK	DINNER	EXERCISE	WATER	
__:___am/pm **WAKE TIME** **Monday** _____ **WEIGHT**	__:___am/pm P1 grain P1 fruit	__:___am/pm P1 fruit	__:___am/pm P1 grain P1 protein P1 fruit P1 veggie	__:___am/pm P1 fruit	__:___am/pm P1 grain P1 protein P1 veggie			**PHASE 1: UNWIND STRESS**
__:___am/pm **WAKE TIME** **Tuesday** _____ **WEIGHT**	__:___am/pm P1 grain P1 fruit	__:___am/pm P1 fruit	__:___am/pm P1 grain P1 protein P1 fruit P1 veggie	__:___am/pm P1 fruit	__:___am/pm P1 grain P1 protein P1 veggie			
__:___am/pm **WAKE TIME** **Wednesday** _____ **WEIGHT**	__:___am/pm P2 protein P2 veggie	__:___am/pm P2 protein	__:___am/pm P2 protein P2 veggie	__:___am/pm P2 protein	__:___am/pm P2 protein P2 veggie			**PHASE 2: UNLOCK FAT STORES**
__:___am/pm **WAKE TIME** **Thursday** _____ **WEIGHT**	__:___am/pm P2 protein P2 veggie	__:___am/pm P2 protein	__:___am/pm P2 protein P2 veggie	__:___am/pm P2 protein	__:___am/pm P2 protein P2 veggie			

	BREAKFAST	SNACK	LUNCH	SNACK	DINNER	EXERCISE	WATER
__:___ am/pm **WAKE TIME** **Friday** _____ **WEIGHT**	__:___ am/pm P3 fruit P3 healthy fat/protein P3 grain P3 veggie	__:___ am/pm P3 veggie P3 healthy fat/protein	__:___ am/pm P3 healthy fat/protein P3 veggie P3 fruit	__:___ am/pm P3 veggie P3 healthy fat/protein	__:___ am/pm P3 healthy fat/protein P3 veggie P3 grain _(optional)		
__:___ am/pm **WAKE TIME** **Saturday** _____ **WEIGHT**	__:___ am/pm P3 fruit P3 healthy fat/protein P3 grain P3 veggie	__:___ am/pm P3 veggie P3 healthy fat/protein	__:___ am/pm P3 healthy fat/protein P3 veggie P3 fruit	__:___ am/pm P3 veggie P3 healthy fat/protein	__:___ am/pm P3 healthy fat/protein P3 veggie P3 grain _(optional)		
__:___ am/pm **WAKE TIME** **Sunday** _____ **WEIGHT**	__:___ am/pm P3 fruit P3 healthy fat/protein P3 grain P3 veggie	__:___ am/pm P3 veggie P3 healthy fat/protein	__:___ am/pm P3 healthy fat/protein P3 veggie P3 fruit	__:___ am/pm P3 veggie P3 healthy fat/protein	__:___ am/pm P3 healthy fat/protein P3 veggie P3 grain _(optional)		

PHASE 3: UNLEASH THE BURN

INDEX

A

apple(s): cinnamon-dusted, 75
   crisp, quick baked, 86
    green apple smoothie, 81
apricot tapioca, 39
Arnold Palmer, 139
artichoke(s): lemon-dressed, 197
   salad, with avocado and
      hearts of palm, 162
asparagus: and bacon salad,
     warm, 114
    bacon-wrapped, 93
    cream of asparagus soup, 174
    and sweet potato soup, 172
avocado: -lime dip, 202
    and shrimp salad, 168
    smoothie, 198
    and tomato toast, 150
    -turkey lettuce wraps, 164

B

bagel: with herbed white bean
     spread, 44
   with smoked salmon, 160
beans. See also chili
    black bean-arugula wrap, 54
    black bean cilantro dip, 83
    five-bean jicama salad, 48
    green, and turkey in lettuce
     cups, 108
    herbed white bean spread, 85
    lemony white bean-dill
     hummus, 194
    and tomato toast, 151
    white bean-dill dip, 84
    wild rice and black bean salad,
     187
beef. See also steak
    baked Italian-style with winter
     veggies, 52
    and cabbage wraps, 66

corned beef and cabbage, 64
Hawaiian burgers, 59
lemon-pepper filet mignon
   and cabbage, 110
mustardy roast beef lettuce
   wraps, 102
roast beef-wrapped pickles,
   131
Southwest-style pot roast, 175
stew, 117
beet and kale smoothie, 200
blackberry sorbet, 205
broccoli: and egg white omelet,
   101
   and fava bean stir-fry, 68
   New York strip with, 125
   and sweet potato sauté, 72
buffalo tip salad, 105
buffalo wrap, 112
burrito: breakfast, 155
   Southwestern, 45
butternut squash soup, 55

C

cacao-coconut ice cream, 203
cacao cookies, 206
cantaloupe smoothie, 82
carrot-orange soup, 57
cashew(s): cashew blackberry
    smoothie, 199
   cashew-quinoa cereal, 150
   chicken, baked, 176
   dip, creamy, 203
cauliflower and leek soup, 171
cereal: brown rice, creamy, 36
   cashew-quinoa, 150
   quinoa, piping hot, 37
   raspberry-studded oatmeal, 157
chicken: baked cashew chicken,
   176
   chicken chili fajita bowl, 181

chicken fajita salad, 106
chicken sausage bowl, 60
coconut, with butternut
   squash, 167
curry, slow-cooked, 166
garlic chicken and vegetables
   over quinoa, 70
lemon-broiled, 109
lemon mustard pepper
   chicken, 123
lettuce wraps, with sweet
   potato hummus, 173
mushroom, and barley soup,
   180
and roasted radish salad,
   177
with shiitakes and mustard
   greens, 115
and sweet potato stew, 51
and veggie kabobs, 116
chili: chicken chili fajita bowl, 181
   four-bean veggie, 188
   vegetarian lentil, 74
chipotle dressing, 144
chocolate-coated cherries, 205
coconut: cacao-coconut ice
   cream, 203
   -cherry smoothie, 198
   coconut almond pudding,
   204
   coconut whipped cream,
   206
   peach-coconut tapioca, 156
cod and veggies, baked, 119
coffee-flavored drink, iced, 200
colon cleanse smoothie, 140
corned beef and cabbage, 64
Cornish game hens: with
    mushroom-quinoa stuffing,
    186
   stuffed, 65

crab salad, 163
cucumber: and sardine canapés, 137
 and tangerine salad, 76
detox smoothie, 141
dips: black bean cilantro, 83
 white bean dill, 84
 chunky mango salsa, 85
 herbed white bean, 85
 southwestern, 144
 avocado-lime, 202
 creamy cashew, 203

D
Dover sole with tomato and brown rice, 67

E
edamame: chopped confetti salad, 104
 and leek salad, 126
 salty, 137
eggplant hummus, 193
eggplant stew, 178
egg(s). *See also* omelet
 benedict, dairy-free, 161
 deviled, 197
 fried, with spinach, 158
 garden egg white scramble, 129
 mustard egg salad, 131
 steak and, 97
 three-pepper egg white soufflé, 130
 whites, hard-boiled, stuffed with minced veggies, 95
exercise, 18, 19, 20, 22, 29

F
Fast Metabolism Diet recap, 12–22
 basics, 12–16
 FAQs, 29–32
 phases, 17–20
 portion sizes, 23–27
 rules, 20–22
fish. *See specific types*
food lists, 89–90, 147–48, 207–8, 213–17

food swaps, 28, 32
freezing meals, 29

G
gazpacho with watermelon chunks, 49
grapefruit with cinnamon, 77
green apple smoothie, 81

H
halibut: and tangerine salad with snow peas and mushrooms, 47
 and veggie stir-fry, 63
Hawaiian burgers, 59
hummus: eggplant, with raw veggies, 193
 lemony white bean-dill, 194
 sweet potato, 173

I
ice cream, cacao-coconut, 203
ice pops, lemon lime, 146

J
jicama: with bacon and lime, 92
 five-bean jicama salad, 48
 minty jicama fruit salad, 78

K
kale chips, 196

L
leek: and cauliflower soup, 171
 and edamame salad, 126
lemon: and lime ice pops, 146
 meringue, 145
 vinaigrette, 143
lemonade, homemade, 140
lentil(s): chili, vegetarian, 74
 ginger-lentil salad, 170
 and veggie stir-fry, 185
lettuce cups, leftover, with dressing, 136
lettuce wrap(s): avocado-turkey, 164
 chicken, with sweet potato hummus, 173
 mustardy roast beef, 102

steak fajita, 120
 steak fajita-avocado, 169
lime: and lemon ice pops, 146
 lime-mint smoothie, 139
 sorbet, 145

M
mango(s): chili-kissed, 76
 salsa, chunky, 85
Master Food List, 213
meal maps, 18, 19, 20, 33
 blanks, 228–35
 samples, 218–27
meal planning, 32–33
meatballs: garden, 134
 Greek, with veggies, 124
meat loaf, turkey: and asparagus, 118
 home-style, 107
meats and poultry. *See specific types*
melon smoothie with mint, 80
meringue: lemon, 145
 rhubarb, 96
minestrone soup, 56
mushroom(s): chicken, and barley soup, 180
 portobellos and mustard greens, 128
 -spinach salad, 191
 and spinach scramble, 94
 tempeh-mushroom hash, 100

O
oatmeal, raspberry-studded, 157
omelet: egg white and broccoli, 101
 spinach-mushroom, 152
orange sorbet, 88
oysters: on cucumbers, 136
 smoked, and cucumbers, 192

P
pancakes: almond berry, 159
 buckwheat flapjacks with blackberry sauce, 38
 oatmeal-almond berry, 154
 sweet potato, 40

papaya with lime juice, 75
pasta and simmered tomato-meat sauce, 69
peach(es): cinnamon, on toast, 37
   -coconut tapioca, 156
   with ginger, 77
   sorbet, 88
pepperoncini dressing, 143
pesto, 202
Phase 1: basics, 17, 18
   food list, 89–90, 213–14
   recipe lists, 35, 210
Phase 2: basics, 17, 19
   food list, 147–48, 214–15
   recipe lists, 91, 211
Phase 3: basics, 17, 19–20
   food list, 207–8, 216–17
   recipe lists, 149, 211–12
pickles, roast beef-wrapped, 131
pineapple, mint grilled, 87
pistachio dressing, 201
pomegranate seeds, spicy, 79
pork: and collard greens, 98
   rosemary pork tenderloin with mustard greens, 121
   spinach salad with squash and, 46
portion sizes, 23–27
portobello mushrooms and mustard greens, 128
pudding, coconut almond, 204
pumpkin cookies, 88
pumpkin-leek soup, 71

Q
quinoa: cereals, 37, 150
   -mushroom stuffing, game hens with, 186
   -pear smoothie, 80
   salad, with radishes and black beans, 189
Quick Guide to Vegetarian and Vegan Recipes, 210

R
raspberry-almond milk smoothie, 199
red bell pepper dressing, 142

rhubarb meringue, 96
rice. See also wild rice
   brown rice cereal, 36
   turkey and veggie fried rice, 182

S
salad(s): artichoke, with avocado and hearts of palm, 162
   asparagus and bacon, warm, 114
   buffalo tip, 105
   chicken fajita, 106
   crab, 163
   cucumber and tangerine, 76
   edamame and leek, 126
   edamame chopped confetti salad, 104
   five-bean jicama, 48
   ginger-lentil, 170
   jicama fruit, minty, 78
   mushroom-spinach, 191
   mustard egg salad, 131
   quinoa, with radishes and black beans, 189
   roasted radish and grilled chicken, 177
   salmon, 165
   sardine, with kale and bacon, 122
   shrimp and avocado, 168
   spinach, with seared pork and squash, 46
   steak, warm, over spinach, 58
   tangerine halibut, with snow peas and mushrooms, 47
   tuna, in endive leaves, 103
   tuna, lemon-dressed, 113
   tuna, red pepper stuffed with, 133
   wild rice and black bean, 187
salad dressing(s):
   tangerine cucumber, 84
   red bell pepper, 142
   pepperoncini, 143
   lemon vinaigrette, 143
   chipotle, 144
   pistachio, 201
   toasted sesame, 201
   pesto, 202

salmon salad, 165
salsa: mango, chunky, 85
   summer, with turkey bacon chips, 135
sardine(s): and cucumber canapés, 137
   and endive cups, 192
   salad, with kale and bacon, 122
   wild sardine pâté, 132
sausage: and cabbage stew, 50
   chicken sausage bowl, 60
shepherd's pie, sweet potato, 62
shrimp: and avocado salad, 168
   and veggie stir-fry, 183
slow cookers, 29, 31
smoked salmon: bagel with, 160
   and celery, 132
   and cucumber, 92
smoothies:
   quinoa pear, 80
   three-melon mint, 80
   green apple, 81
   tropical, 83
   cantaloupe, 82
   lime-mint, 139
   colon cleanse, 140
   detox, 141
   avocado, 198
   coconut-cherry, 198
   raspberry almond milk, 199
   cashew blackberry, 199
   beet and kale, 200
smoothies, 22, 30
   Phase 1, 80–82
   Phase 2, 139–41
   Phase 3, 198–200
sorbet: blackberry, 205
   lime, 145
   orange, 88
   peach, 88
   strawberry-beet, 87
soup(s). See also chili; stew
   asparagus and sweet potato, 172
   butternut squash, 55
   chicken, mushroom, and barley, 180
   cream of asparagus, 174

gazpacho, 49
gingered carrot-orange, 57
ginger pumpkin-leek, 71
leek and cauliflower, 171
minestrone, 56
Southwestern dip, fiery, 144
soy foods, 21, 32
spinach: burrito with bacon and, 45
fried egg with, 158
-mushroom omelet, 152
-mushroom salad, 191
and mushroom scramble, 94
salad, with seared pork and squash, 46
steak. *See also* beef
and eggs, 97
mustard-coated, broiled, 111
New York strip with broccoli, 125
salad, warm, over spinach, 58
steak fajita-avocado lettuce wrap, 169
steak fajita lettuce wrap, 120
stew. *See also* chili; soup(s)
beef, 117
chicken and sweet potato, 51
eggplant, 178
sausage and cabbage, 50
tempeh vegetable, 127
stir-fry: broccoli and fava bean, 68
gingered shrimp and veggie, 183
halibut and veggie, 63

lentil and veggie, 185
Southwestern breakfast, 99
strawberry-beet sorbet, 87
sun tea mojito, 141
sweet potato: and asparagus soup, 172
and broccoli sauté, 72
and chicken stew, 51
fries, oven-baked, 195
hummus, 173
pancakes, 40
shepherd's pie, 62

T
tangerine-cucumber dressing, 84
tapioca: apricot, 39
peach-coconut, 156
tea, 31
Arnold Palmer, 139
sun tea mojito, 141
tempeh-mushroom hash, 100
tempeh vegetable stew, 127
toast: avocado and tomato, 150
black bean and tomato, 151
cinnamon peaches on, 37
toasted sesame dressing, 201
tofu jerky, peppery, 138
tostada, 61
tropical smoothie, 82
tuna: melt, tomato-topped, 153
salad, in endive leaves, 103
salad, lemon-dressed, 113
salad, red pepper stuffed with, 133

and veggie sandwich, tangy, 43
turkey: -avocado lettuce wrap, 164
and bell pepper rice, 190
burgers, with sweet potatoes, 184
ground, green beans and, in lettuce cups, 108
meat loaf, and asparagus, 118
meat loaf, home-style, 107
Mediterranean, with wild rice, 53
sloppy Joe wrap, 42
smoked turkey-vegetable hash, 179
and veggie fried rice, 182

V
vegetable curry, 73
vegetables, 24, 27, 30–31
vegetarians and vegans, 21, 28, 32
recipe list, 210–12

W
water, 20, 31
watermelon with mint, 79
wild rice: and black bean salad, 187
patties, spicy Southwest, 41
wrap(s). *See also* lettuce wrap(s)
beef and cabbage, 66
black bean-arugula, 54
buffalo wrap, 112
sloppy Joe turkey, 42

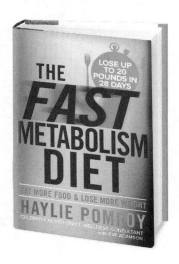
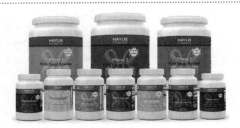
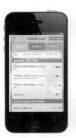